Chair Yoga for Weight Loss

Complete, Easy-to-Follow Guide for Seniors Over 60 to
Slim Down, Boost Energy, Feel Younger and Healthier in
Just 10 Minutes a Day – Includes 14-Day Challenge

Kate M. Right

Contents

Introduction

Welcome! This book is your clear pathway to losing weight and revitalizing both your body and spirit through the joy and simplicity of chair yoga—a practice thoughtfully designed for your unique needs and lifestyle.

The journey of chair yoga began in 1982 when visionary yoga teacher Lakshmi Voelker developed chair-based poses specifically for students with arthritis and mobility limitations. Since then, chair yoga has evolved and gained widespread popularity for its accessibility and modified approach to traditional yoga. It is especially beneficial for seniors, providing gentle yet effective movement to enhance fitness and well-being.

Let's Be Honest

While numerous chair yoga books exist for seniors, many may leave you feeling overwhelmed or unmotivated by complex illustrations and video guides that disrupt the flow of your exercise routine. Chair yoga isn't just about physical activity; it's about reclaiming control over your health and, more importantly, rediscovering joy and vitality. This guide provides a practical, easy-to-follow approach, enabling you to enjoy the benefits of chair yoga daily without the hassle of complicated instructions or technological interruptions.

What Sets This Book Apart?

Drawing on my experiences as a fitness and wellness advocate and inspired by my published Amazon Best Sellers, such as *Simplified Chair Yoga for Seniors Over 60* and *Weight Loss Hacks for Women Over 40*, I have crafted this guide with the senior community in mind. Having supported my active grandparents and worked closely with senior communities, I understand the importance of simplicity in creating healthy and sustainable routines. My goal is to make weight loss through chair yoga enjoyable and seamlessly integrated into your daily life, offering a gentle path to enhanced health and well-being.

Efficient and Effective - Just 10 Minutes a Day

Through extensive research, daily practice, and coaching seniors, I have curated a set of 22 essential poses focused on weight loss and targeted toning. I've also handpicked 10 poses for stretching and relaxation that you will find effective in relieving tension, muscle pain, or joint pain. By dedicating just 10 minutes a day, you can improve mobility, posture, balance, and flexibility, all while losing weight. Through consistent practice, you'll feel lighter, more energetic, and increasingly independent, showing that age is just a number.

Easy to Follow - Large and Simple Illustrations

Each chair yoga pose comes with large, clear illustrations and concise instructions to ensure a stress-free learning experience. My focus is on the essentials, guiding you through each pose with confidence and ease, using illustrations that highlight the final state or essential steps, thereby preventing you from feeling overwhelmed.

100% Seat-Based for Maximum Comfort and Safety

The carefully selected chair yoga poses prioritize comfort and safety, allowing practice entirely from your chair. This approach alleviates the difficulty of constant movement during exercise, helping you increase metabolism, burn calories, and build strength regardless of your current level of mobility.

Easy to Remember — Enjoyable and Sustainable Routines

These poses will become second nature over time, blending effortlessly into daily life and proving that fitness can be both fun and sustainable.

Suitable for All Fitness Levels

This guide is adaptable for all fitness levels. From basic poses to variations with increased intensity, it offers a safe, gentle routine that evolves with you.

Holistic Approach — Additional Health & Wellness Tips

Beyond chair yoga, you'll discover valuable tips for holistic wellness, including nutrition hacks, herbal remedies, improved sleep, mental well-being practices, and increased mobility that collectively and efficiently support weight loss and long-term health. These strategies complement and work in harmony with your chair yoga routine to boost energy, confidence, and joy.

Whether you're new to chair yoga or seeking a streamlined routine, this guide is designed to be easy, enjoyable, and effective. Let's embark on this rewarding journey together—achieving sustainable weight loss while having fun and enhancing your overall physical and mental well-being.

Chapter 1:

Get Ready for Chair Yoga

How to Use This Book?

Understand Benefits and Try 22 Weight Loss Poses

In this guide, I've handpicked 22 chair yoga poses that work well together to help lose weight and tone the body with visible results. I've broken down each pose with benefits, step-by-step instructions, and precautionary tips (when applicable). Understanding the benefits of each pose allows you to concentrate on the ones that matter most to you. While some benefits—like relieving tension or improving circulation—may overlap, don't skip the details. Each pose targets different muscles, tendons, and joints, so practicing each one will help you improve your overall mobility and strength. The precautionary tips are there to help you stay safe and avoid common mistakes.

Try 10 Stretching and Relaxation Poses

I included 10 basic and highly effective poses to help you stretch and relax. You can use these as a subset or a complete set of those poses at any time of the day. It's entirely up to you how you want to incorporate them into your daily movements. You can do these poses either before or after your weight loss chair yoga routine any time you feel tension. These poses do increase dopamine levels!

Do the 14-Day Challenge to Practice Mixed Routines

After you try each pose in the order they're listed, you can start the 14-Day Challenge I've carefully designed. This progressive approach provides ample time to build muscle memory, mix up the poses to keep your routine fun and boost your metabolism. Doing the same exercise without variations can cause your metabolism to plateau. In my weight loss books, as noted in the Introduction and References, I explain why shorter, varied routines are often more effective for weight loss and long-term management. Repeating the same workout can lead to metabolic adaptation, reducing calorie burn. Varying movement intensity and sequencing helps prevent plateaus, keeps the body challenged, and supports a more active metabolism.

Repeat or Create Your Sequence of Poses

By the time you finish the 14-Day Challenge, you'll master these poses. From there, you can repeat the 14-Day Challenge or select poses of your choice for a quick 10-minute daily routine.

Integrate Additional Health and Wellness Tips

Be sure to incorporate my additional yet simple health and wellness tips on eating, sleeping, mental wellness, and mobility. This holistic approach will help you feel even more energetic and confident.

Now you understand how to use this book, let's go over the essential items to prepare you for chair yoga.

Preparation Essentials

What Kind of Chair to Use

Use a sturdy, movable chair with a flat seat, no wheels, and no side arms. I say movable because you want to place the chair in an area with no blockage on the front, left, and right sides. A couch or a sofa is technically a chair, but it's not generally movable and has rest arms. Also, ensure the chair is placed on a flat, solid surface to prevent wobbling as you transition from one pose to another.

What to Wear

You can wear pajamas, sweatshirts, pants, t-shirts, and trousers that are not too tight, as you will be lifting and extending your legs, as well as extending and swinging your arms. You will press your feet onto the floor to help you stay balanced. If you wear socks, ensure they don't slide. If you wear shoes, make sure you wear flat shoes.

Breathing Basics

Breathing is a crucial aspect of chair yoga, enabling you to relax, focus on your poses, and unite your body and mind. There are many fancy breathing terms. I will keep it simple for you. In short, try to breathe deeper than usual and focus on your breath as your body moves. Now, let's practice a few deep breaths together.

You can try two basic breathing techniques, which you can use before starting and at the end of your routine to help you relax and calm your mind:

1. **Diaphragmatic Breathing (Belly Breathing)**
   - Find a Comfortable Position – Sit down in a relaxed posture.
   - Place Hands for Awareness (Optional) – Put one hand on the chest and the other on the belly. Note: This optional hand placement is only for practice to help you distinguish between deep and shallow breathing.
   - Inhale Deeply Through the Nose – Breathe in slowly, allowing the belly to rise while keeping the chest still.
   - Exhale Slowly Through the Mouth – Let the belly fall as air is released gently through pursed lips.
   - Repeat – Continue for several breaths, maintaining a steady, slow rhythm. This technique promotes relaxation and helps reduce tension.

2. **Equal Breathing**
   - Find a Comfortable Position – Sit down with a straight spine.
   - Inhale Through the Nose – Breathe in slowly, counting to four.
   - Exhale Through the Nose – Breathe out for the same count of four.
   - Maintain a Steady Rhythm – Continue inhaling and exhaling for equal counts.

- Adjust as Needed – Increase the count (e.g., to six or eight) for deeper relaxation. Maintain steady, even breaths to promote calmness and balance.

Next, practice breathing with movement. Synchronize your breath, using either breathing technique with the flow of poses:

- Inhale during upward or expansive movements (e.g., reaching arms up).
- Exhale during downward or contracting movements (e.g., folding forward or turning your upper body).

Don't worry about being precise when you count how long you hold your breath. Whatever feels comfortable is fine. Inhaling or exhaling for a count of 4 or 5 is perfectly fine. As you increase your cardio fitness, you will find deeper breathing easier. People with better cardio fitness often have greater lung capacity and improved oxygen exchange efficiency, allowing them to inhale and exhale for a longer count. Please don't force yourself to hold your breath longer than you can.

When Is the Best Time to Do Chair Yoga

The beauty of chair yoga is that you can do it anytime! I don't recommend doing it before bedtime, as it may increase your heart rate and affect your sleep. Once you complete the 14-Day Challenge and have a good understanding of the benefits of each pose, you can do stretches whenever you feel tension in your body. You can do the more rigorous poses when you are alert and energetic. It's best to set aside a specific time each day for a quick

10-minute routine to turn it into a long-term habit. I highly recommend starting your day with this fitness routine to set a high note! If you like to repeat a session in the afternoon, go for it.

Stay Hydrated

If you do chair yoga first thing in the morning, you may not feel like eating breakfast, but make sure to hydrate before you start. You don't need to drink excessively right before each session, but a little water before your session goes a long way! Hydration improves muscle function, keeps joints flexible, and supports blood flow.

Once you have your chair ready and practice the breathing techniques a couple of times, all that's left is to drink some water before you start. It's that simple!

Reminders

For those familiar with chair yoga, this book doesn't reinvent the wheel. It's about making chair yoga simpler and more enjoyable for seniors so you can easily incorporate it into your daily routine. Keep an open mind and follow the 14-Day Challenge to experience the benefits firsthand.

Always consult a healthcare provider before starting any new exercise regimen, especially if you have any pre-existing health conditions.

Next, let's dive into the 22 essential poses I've carefully selected to simplify your weight loss journey through chair yoga.

Chapter 2: Full-Body Activation & Metabolism Boost

F1. Seated Mountain

Benefits:

1. **Improves Posture:** Encourages proper spinal alignment, helping to prevent slouching and promote an upright posture.
2. **Enhances Awareness:** Increases body awareness and mindfulness by bringing attention to breath, alignment, and the present moment.
3. **Strengthens Core Muscles:** Engages the core muscles during this pose supports stability and balance.
4. **Promotes Relaxation:** Aids in calming the mind and reducing stress, making it an excellent grounding exercise.
5. **Accessible Alignment Practice:** Suitable for individuals of all fitness levels, offering a gentle introduction to yoga fundamentals.

Instructions:

- Sit up straight with feet flat on the floor, hip-width apart.
- Root your feet into the ground.
- Root your sitting bones into the chair.

- Lengthen your head toward the ceiling to create a neutral spine, engage your core and lengthen your spine, imagining a string pulling the top of your head upwards.
- Extend your arms up, away from your ears, with your palms together.
- Keep your fingers soft and pointed up.
- Hold the pose for a few breaths.
- Drop your arms and relax your shoulders.

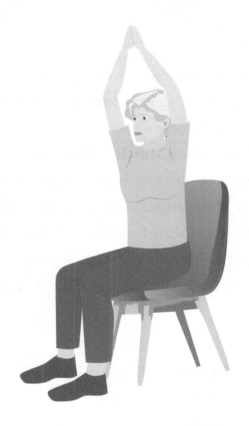

F2. Seated Warrior 1

Benefits:

1. **Strengthens Legs**: Engages and strengthens the quadriceps, hamstrings, and calves, promoting lower body strength.

2. **Opens Hips**: Stretches and opens the hip flexors, which can become tight from prolonged sitting.

3. **Improves Balance**: Encourages better balance and stability through engagement of the core and lower body muscles.

4. **Enhances Focus and Concentration**: Holding the pose requires mental focus, helping to improve concentration.

5. **Encourages Proper Alignment**: Promotes good posture and alignment, supporting overall body awareness.

Instructions:

- Sit sideways near the edge of the chair with feet flat on the floor, facing right.

- Extend your left leg back with toes on the floor; bend the front knee.

- Raise your arms upwards or leave your hands on your lap if needed.

- Hold for a few breaths, then switch sides.

- Sit sideways near the edge of the chair with feet flat on the floor, facing left.

- Extend your right leg back with toes on the floor; bend the front knee.

- Raise your arms upwards or leave your hands on your lap if needed.

- Hold for a few breaths, then return to center.

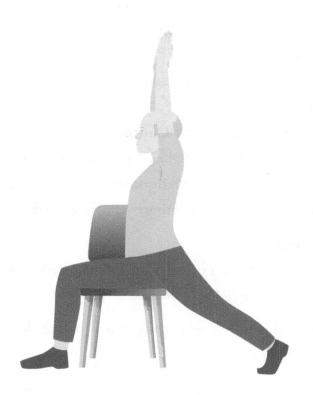

F3. Seated Warrior 2

Benefits:

1. **Strengthens Legs and Arms**: Engages and builds muscle strength in the legs, arms, and core.
2. **Improves Flexibility**: Enhances flexibility in the hips and inner thighs.
3. **Promotes Balance and Stability**: Encourages balance and a stable posture.
4. **Accessible Exercise**: Suitable for individuals with mobility concerns or those who prefer seated workouts.

Instructions:

- Sit sideways on a sturdy chair with your right side aligned with the chair's backrest. Ensure your right thigh is parallel to the chair seat and your feet are firmly planted on the ground.
- Extend your left leg to the side, keeping it straight, while your right leg remains bent at a 90-degree angle. Make sure both feet are flat on the ground, with the right foot facing forward and the left foot slightly turned. If keeping your left foot fully flat is uncomfortable, press firmly into the ball of your foot for stability.
- Stretch your arms out to the sides parallel to the floor, aligning them with your shoulders. Your fingertips should be active, extending in opposite directions.

- Keep your torso upright, facing toward the bent right knee. Engage your core to maintain balance and stability.
- Turn your head to gaze over your right fingertips, maintaining a relaxed neck and shoulders.
- Hold this position for several breaths, focusing on the stretch and engaging your muscles. Feel the stretch in your inner thighs and the strengthening of your core and arms.
- Gently release the pose and switch sides, repeating with your left knee bent.

Precautions:
- Depending on the length of your legs and the height of the chair, the foot extended behind can have varied positions, either pointing forward and using the ball of the foot to firmly press the ground. Or slightly turn the foot, so you can have your entire foot flat on the ground. Do whatever that makes your ankle comfortable, while serving the purpose of stretching your leg.

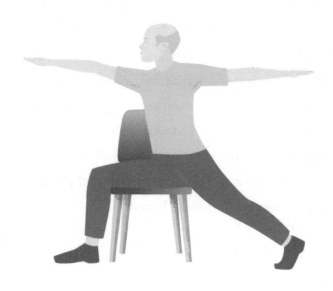

F4. Chair Crescent Lunge

Benefits:

1. **Improves hip mobility**, especially for tight hip flexors
2. **Stretches thighs, groin, and abdomen.**
3. **Opens the chest and strengthens the back.**
4. **Enhances balance** while safely seated.
5. **Engages the core** gently, promoting stability.
6. **Boosts circulation** and oxygen flow.

Instructions:

- Sit sideways on the chair. Position your right hip facing the chair's backrest. Keep both feet flat on the floor.

- Slide the right leg back. Extend your right leg behind you. Keep the toes tucked under or flat on the floor, depending on your flexibility. Your left knee stays bent at 90°, directly over the left ankle.
- Square your hips forward as much as possible. Lengthen the spine. Sit tall and avoid arching your back.
- Reach your arms upward with palms facing each other. Keep your shoulders relaxed and down.
- Engage the core. Pull your navel toward the spine. Stay in this position for 3–5 slow breaths.

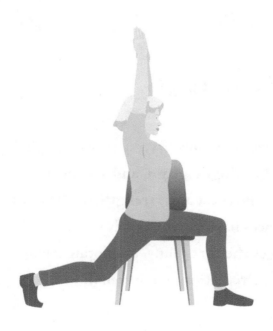

- Turn your torso to face the chair's backrest. Extend your arms outward and hold for 2-3 slow breaths.

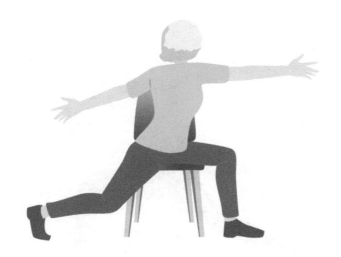

- Turn your torso, facing forward. Place your hands together in front of your chest, while keeping the right leg extended. Hold in this position for 2-3 slow breaths.

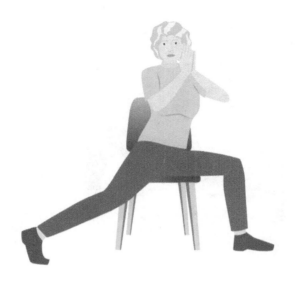

- Lower and relax your arms. Bring the right leg back to the center and face forward.
- Repeat on the other side. Follow the same steps with left leg extended behind you.

F5. Seated Jumping Jacks

Benefits:

1. **Increases heart rate** to support cardiovascular health
2. **Improves coordination** between upper and lower body
3. **Enhances circulation and oxygen flow**
4. **Strengthens arms, legs, and core** with repeated motion
5. **Boosts energy and mood** through light aerobic activity

Instructions:

- Sit tall in a sturdy chair. Keep your feet flat on the floor and core lightly engaged.

- Sit toward the front edge of the chair, keeping your spine long.

- Place your arms at your sides and feet together.

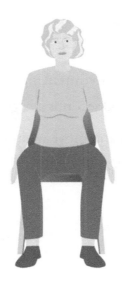

- Raise your arms overhead in a wide "V" shape. At the same time, step your feet out wide to the sides.

- Lower your arms back to your sides and step your feet back together.

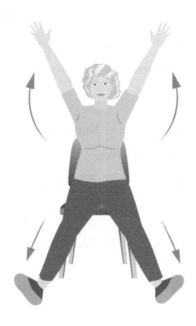

- Repeat at a steady rhythm. Aim for 8–12 repetitions, or continue for 30–60 seconds at a gentle pace

- Breathe naturally and move within your comfort range.

F6. Seated Kick Punches

Benefits:

1. **Full-Body Activation**: Engages arms, legs, and core — improving overall muscle tone and coordination.
2. **Boosts Cardiovascular Health**: Elevates heart rate gently, promoting circulation and heart health without strain.
3. **Improves Balance & Stability**: Builds leg and core strength, helping reduce the risk of falls and improving everyday movement.
4. **Enhances Coordination**: Stimulates brain-body connection, supporting cognitive sharpness.
5. **Promotes Weight Loss**: Increases calorie burn through compound movement.

Instructions:

- Lift your **right leg** off the floor.
- At the same time, punch your **left arm** across your body (diagonally toward the right)
- Keep your back straight — don't lean.
- Return to start — Gently lower your leg and arm back to the starting position.
- Breathe naturally — exhale as you punch/kick, inhale as you return. Start slow and build a steady rhythm.
- Switch sides — Lift your left leg and punch your right arm forward.

- Keep alternating sides: right kick + left punch, then left kick + right punch.

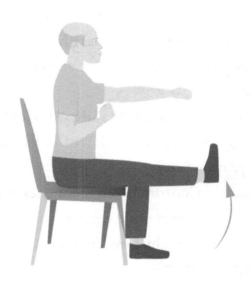

Chapter 3 - Core & Waist Toning

C1. Seated Hip Circles

This pose focuses on improving mobility and flexibility in the hips, pelvis, and lower back. This pose targets the hip flexors, glutes, and lumbar spine, providing a gentle massage for the lower back and pelvic region.

Benefits:

1. **Improves Hip Mobility and Flexibility:** Gently lubricates the hip joints. Increases range of motion in the hip sockets. Helps loosen tight hip flexors and glutes from prolonged sitting.

2. **Enhances Lower Back Support:** Engages the lower back muscles in a controlled, safe way. Reduces stiffness and tension in the lumbar spine.

3. **Strengthens Core and Postural Muscles:** Encourages gentle engagement of abdominal and oblique muscles. Activates the muscles that stabilize the pelvis.

4. **Supports Circulation and Lymphatic Flow:** Stimulates blood flow to the pelvis and legs. Aids lymphatic drainage in the lower body. Helps reduce swelling or stagnation from sedentary behavior.

Instructions:

- Sit on a sturdy chair with your feet flat on the floor, hip-width apart. Sit upright with your back straight and shoulders relaxed.
- Engage your abdominal muscles to support your lower back during the movement.
- Slowly shift your torso forward, moving in a circular motion to the right.
- Lean your torso to the right, then circle it back, rounding through the lower back.
- Continue the circle to the left and return to the starting position.
- Keep the movement slow and smooth, creating a rhythmic flow.
- Repeat: Complete 5-10 circles in one direction, then reverse the direction for an equal number of circles.
- Breathe mindfully. Inhale as you circle forward and exhale as you round back.
- Return to an upright position and take a few deep breaths before moving on.

Precautions:

This pose is perfect as a warm-up or a stress-relieving stretch during a long day of sitting. Take these tips into consideration.

- Keep the motion gentle to avoid straining your lower back.

- Adjust the size of the circles based on your comfort level and flexibility.
- For a deeper stretch, emphasize leaning forward and back during the motion.

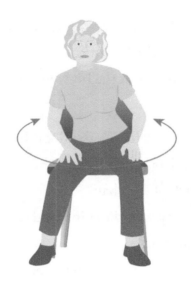

C2. Seated Torso Twist

Benefits:

1. **Improves Spinal Mobility**: The twisting motion helps maintain and improve the spine's range of motion, essential for daily movements and overall back health.
2. **Aids Digestion**: Twisting poses can stimulate the digestive organs, promoting better digestion and detoxification.

3. **Enhances Posture**: Regular practice can help align the spine and improve posture, particularly for those who spend long hours sitting.
4. **Releases Tension**: It helps release tension in the back and shoulders, providing a gentle stretch that can relieve stress.
5. **Increases Blood Flow**: The twisting action encourages circulation, which can aid in delivering nutrients and oxygen throughout the body more efficiently.

Instructions:

- Sit tall with feet flat on the floor, hip-width apart.
- Place your left hand on the right knee and your right hand on the back of the chair.
- Inhale to lengthen the spine, and exhale to twist your torso to the right gently.
- Hold for a few breaths, then repeat on the other side.

For a more advanced version, place your left hand on the right edge of your seat, your right hand on the back of the chair, and turn your upper body and neck more. Repeat the same on the other side. You should feel your core tightening as you twist.

Precautions:

- Gradually increase how much you turn your upper body.
- Remember to breathe!

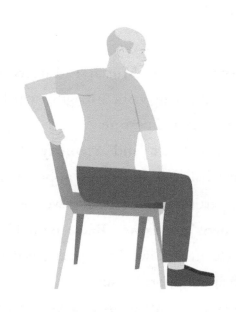

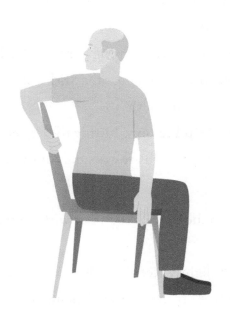

33

C3. Chair Boat Pose

Benefits:

1. **Strengthens Core Muscles:** Targets the abdominal muscles, enhancing core strength, which is crucial for overall stability and posture.
2. **Improves Balance and Stability:** Engages the core, maintains balance, and helps improve overall stability, which is particularly beneficial as we age.
3. **Strengthens the Lower Back:** By holding the posture, the muscles in the lower back get engaged, helping to build strength and support the spine.
4. **Enhances Concentration and Focus:** Balancing in this pose requires concentration, helping to sharpen focus and mental clarity.
5. **Supports Posture:** A strong core and back contribute to better posture, reducing the risk of back pain and promoting spinal health.
6. **Tones the Hip Flexors:** Lifting the legs engages and tones the hip flexors, which are essential for mobility.

Instructions:

- Sit closer to the edge of the chair with your knees bent and feet flat.
- Lean back slightly, keeping your back straight.
- Lift your feet off the floor, balancing on your sit bones.

- Keep your arms parallel to the floor or hold the sides of the chair for support.
- Hold for a few breaths, then lower your feet.
- This pose is more advanced than the Seated Leg Lift because you raise both legs using more core muscles. An even more advanced variation is lifting your lower legs to parallel the floor, which tightens your midsection even more.

Precautions:
- Hold tight to the two sides of the chair to prevent your body from slipping.
- You might feel your core and legs shake as you try to use your core muscles. If uncomfortable, keep your lower legs at an angle, not parallel to the floor, until your core muscle is strong enough.

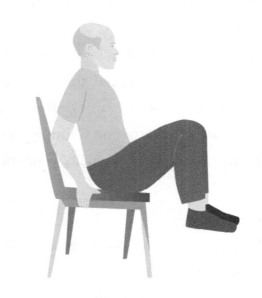

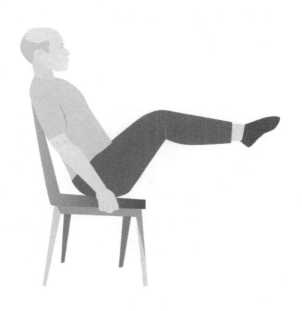

C4. Seated Forward Bend

Benefits:

1. **Stretches the Back and Hamstrings**: Provides a deep stretch to the spine and the muscles at the back of the legs, helping alleviate tension and increase flexibility.
2. **Calms the Mind**: The forward folding motion encourages relaxation, which can help reduce stress and promote mental clarity.
3. **Improves Flexibility**: Regular practice enhances flexibility in the back and legs, promoting a greater range of motion.
4. **Aids Digestion**: The folding position gently compresses the abdomen, which can help stimulate digestive processes.
5. **Enhances Posture**: Encourages spinal lengthening and proper alignment, supporting better overall posture.

Instructions:

- Sit tall with feet flat on the floor.
- Inhale, lengthen your spine.
- Exhale, hinge at the hips, and lean forward, reaching your hands towards your feet.
- Hold gently for a few deep breaths, then slowly rise back.

Precautions:

- Gradually increase how far you can bend forward.

- Slowly lift your head and spine, and avoid a sudden upward lift.

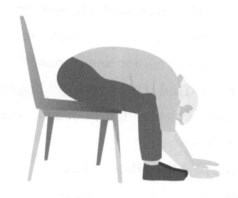

C5. Chair Side Bend

Benefits:

1. **Tones Oblique Muscles:** Effectively works the side abdominal muscles, helping to tone and strengthen the obliques.

2. **Enhances Core Strength:** By engaging the core, this pose strengthens the abdominal area overall, supporting balance and stability.

3. **Improves Flexibility:** The bending motion increases flexibility in the sides of the body, promoting a greater range of motion.

4. **Promotes Better Posture:** Strengthening the core muscles aids in maintaining proper posture, reducing strain on the back and neck.

5. **Stimulates Digestion:** Gentle lateral bends can help stimulate the digestive organs by massaging the abdominal area.

6. **Relieves Tension**: The stretch provided by side bends can release tension in the lower back and sides, relieving stiffness.

Instructions:

- Sit straight on a chair with both feet flat on the ground, hip-width apart.
- Place your right hand behind your head and your left hand on your hip or down by your side.
- Inhale to prepare; as you exhale, bend your torso to the left, bringing your right elbow towards your left side.
- Keep your chest open and core engaged.
- Inhale to return to the upright position.
- Repeat for several repetitions, then switch to the other side.

Note: This pose sounds similar to the Seated Side Stretch, which is often slower and more focused on gently lengthening the side body. In contrast, Chair Side Bend involves a more active engagement of the core to help tone the sides of the body (obliques). Both poses are beneficial for improving flexibility and strength, but they serve slightly different purposes in a yoga routine.

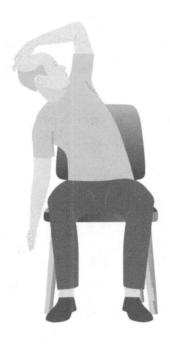

C6. Seated Marching

Benefits:

1. **Enhances Cardiovascular Health**: Increases the heart rate, promoting improved cardiovascular fitness even while seated.
2. **Strengthens Core Muscles**: Engages the core, helping to build strength and stability in the abdominal area.

3. **Improves Leg Strength and Mobility**: Strengthens the hip flexors and leg muscles, enhancing overall mobility and flexibility.

4. **Boosts Coordination and Balance**: Alternating knee lifts require coordination, which helps improve balance and motor skills.

5. **Promotes Circulation**: The rhythmic movement enhances blood flow throughout the body, which is beneficial for overall health.

6. **Accessible Exercise**: This pose is accessible as it can be performed by individuals with varied fitness levels, making it suitable for seniors or those with mobility issues.

Instructions:

- Sit tall with feet flat on the floor.
- Alternate lifting each knee towards your chest as if marching.
- Keep your core engaged throughout the movement.
- Increase the speed gradually for a cardiovascular effect.

It's up to you how long or how fast you want to march. You can start with marching for 1 minute and gradually increase your time on this exercise to get a mini cardio workout.

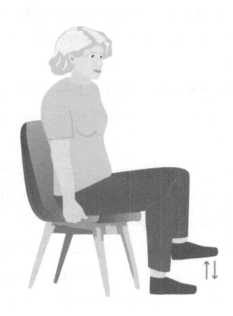

C7. Seated Bicycle Crunches

Benefits:

1. **Strengthens Core Muscles:** This pose effectively targets the entire core, including the upper and lower abdominals, enhancing overall core strength.

2. **Tones Obliques:** The twisting motion in this exercise specifically engages the oblique muscles on the sides of the abdomen, aiding in muscle toning.

3. **Improves Flexibility and Mobility:** The side-to-side motion helps increase flexibility and mobility in the torso and lower back.

4. **Enhances Coordination and Balance:** Performing bicycle crunches while seated requires coordination, contributing to improved balance and motor skills.

5. **Supports Posture:** A strong core is essential for good posture, and this exercise helps develop the muscles needed to maintain proper alignment.

6. **Accessible and Low-Impact:** Because it is performed in a seated position, it is accessible to individuals with different fitness levels or mobility issues and those who prefer low-impact exercises.

Instructions:

- Sit near the edge of a sturdy chair with feet flat on the floor. Keep the back straight and core engaged.
- Place hands lightly behind the head for support.
- Lift the right knee toward the chest while gently twisting the upper body to bring the left elbow toward the right knee. Keep the movement slow and controlled.
- Lower the right foot back to the floor and return to the starting position.
- Lift the left knee toward the chest while twisting the right elbow toward the left knee.
- Continue alternating sides in a steady, pedaling motion, keeping the core engaged.
- Focus on slow, controlled movements and deep breathing.
- Progress at Your Own Pace: Gradually increase speed for a light cardio effect.

It's up to you how many repetitions or how fast you want to do these crunches. Start with 10 repetitions and gradually increase your time on this exercise to get a mini cardio workout.

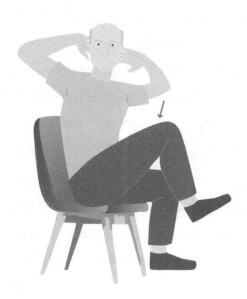

C8. Prayer Twist

Benefits:

1. **Improves spinal flexibility** and posture.
2. **Enhances core strength** and stability.
3. **Aids digestion** and detoxification.
4. **Reduces back and shoulder tension**.

Instructions:

- Sit tall on a sturdy chair with feet hip-width apart and flat on the floor. Knees are directly over ankles.

- Lengthen your spine upwards, sitting as tall as possible.
- Place your palms together at your chest in a prayer position.
- On your exhale, engage your core and gently twist your torso to the right.
- Hook your left elbow outside your right knee for a deeper twist, pressing palms together.
- Hold the twist for 3–5 breaths, maintaining a long spine. Gaze over your right shoulder if comfortable.

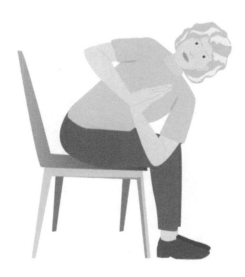

- Inhale and slowly return to center. Repeat on the left side, hooking your right elbow outside your left knee.

- Return to neutral, take a few deep breaths, and notice the effects.

Chapter 4 – Legs, Glutes & Thigh Toning

L1. Seated Knee Lifts

Benefits:

1. **Strengthens Core Muscles**: By lifting the knees, this pose targets the lower abdominal muscles, helping to build core strength.

2. **Enhances Hip Flexor Flexibility and Strength:** It works the hip flexors, promoting flexibility and strength in these essential muscles used in many daily activities.

3. **Improves Balance and Stability:** Strengthens the core, contributing to better overall balance and stability; this is crucial for daily movements and preventing falls, especially in seniors.

4. **Tones the Lower Body:** Helps tone the thighs and improve muscle control in the lower body.

5. **Supports Better Posture**: A strong core is vital for maintaining good posture, reducing strain on the back, and improving overall alignment.

Instructions:

- Sit tall with feet flat on the floor.
- Lift one knee towards your chest, engaging your core.
- Hold for a moment, then lower it back down.

- Alternate legs, performing the movement in a controlled manner.
- The longer you hold, the more you're exercising your core muscles. Be sure to breathe in and out.

Precautions:
- Don't hold your breath.
- Gradually increase how high and how fast you lift your knees.

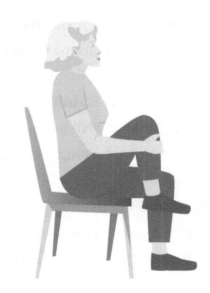

L2. Seated Leg Lifts

Benefits:

1. **Strengthens Leg Muscles**: Targets the quadriceps and hip flexors, helping to build strength in the legs.
2. **Engages Core Muscles**: Involves the abdominal muscles, especially when holding the leg in an elevated position, contributing to core stability and strength.
3. **Improves Flexibility**: Enhances flexibility in the hip joints and promotes a greater range of motion.
4. **Supports Balance and Stability**: By strengthening the lower body and core, this pose aids in maintaining better balance and stability, which is essential for daily activities.
5. **Accessible Exercise**: This can be performed by individuals at various fitness levels, making it a versatile addition to chair yoga routines.

Instructions:

- Sit tall and grip the sides of the chair.
- Lift one leg straight out in front of you and hold for 3-4 slow breaths.
- Lower the leg and repeat with the other leg.

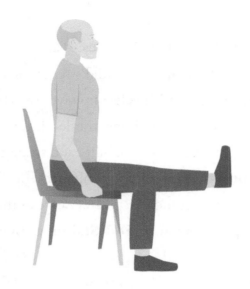

L3. Seated Hamstring Stretch with Core Hold

Benefits:

1. **Engages the core** to support lower back health.
2. **Improves posture** and spinal alignment.
3. **Enhances flexibility** in the legs while seated.
4. **Supports balance** and muscular control.

Instructions:

- Sit upright on a sturdy chair, feet flat on the floor, spine tall.
- Extend one leg forward, straightening the knee as much as possible, heel resting on the floor with toes pointing up.

- Engage the core by gently drawing the navel toward the spine.
- Place hands on the opposite thigh or rest gently on the sides of the extended leg (avoid pushing on the knee).
- Hinge forward slightly from the hips, keeping the back flat and long. Avoid rounding the spine.
- Hold this stretch while keeping the core engaged. Breathe slowly and steadily.
- Stay in this position for 3–5 deep breaths. Feel the stretch in the back of the extended leg while maintaining a stable, active core.
- Return to upright, bend the extended leg, and place the foot flat.
- Repeat on the other side.

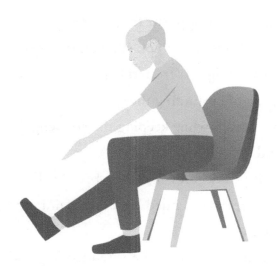

L4. Chair Tree

This pose focuses on enhancing balance, strengthening the lower body, and improving core stability.

Benefits:

1. **Improves Balance**: This pose helps enhance balance and stability, crucial for daily movements and fall prevention.
2. **Strengthens Core and Legs**: Engages the core muscles and strengthens the legs, supporting overall stability and posture.
3. **Enhances Focus and Concentration**: Maintaining the balance needed in this pose can improve mental focus and concentration.

4. **Promotes Flexibility**: Gently stretches the inner thighs and hips, contributing to greater flexibility.

Instructions:

- Sit tall, keep your feet flat and spine straight.
- Place your right foot on your left knee.
- Engage your core, and focus on a point ahead.
- Hands in prayer at the chest or overhead.
- Maintain for several breaths, then switch sides.

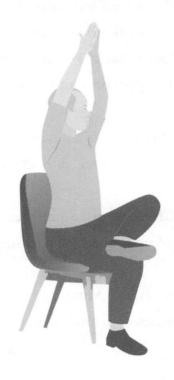

Chapter 5: Arms, Shoulders & Back Toning

U1. Seated Eagle Arms

Benefits:

1. **Enhances Shoulder Flexibility**: Stretches the shoulders, helping to increase flexibility and range of motion.
2. **Releases Upper Back Tension**: Alleviates tension and stiffness in the upper back and neck, relieving stress-related tightness.
3. **Improves Posture**: Encourages proper alignment by opening the upper back and chest, promoting better posture.
4. **Increases Circulation**: Stimulates blood flow to the shoulders and upper back, supporting muscle health and recovery.
5. **Strengthens Arm Muscles**: Engages the arm and shoulder muscles, contributing to upper body strength.

Instructions:

- Sit with feet flat on the floor.
- Cross your right arm under the left, wrapping at the elbows.
- Try to bring palms together or as close as possible.

- Lift elbows slightly and hold for a few breaths, then switch arms.
- Cross your left arm under the right, wrapping at the elbows.
- Try to bring palms together or as close as possible.
- Lift elbows slightly and hold for a few breaths.

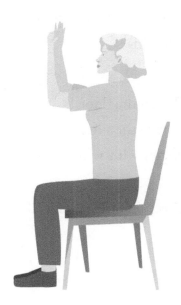

U2. Seated Arm Circles

Benefits:

1. **Increases Shoulder Mobility**: Rotating the arms helps to enhance the range of motion in the shoulder joints, promoting flexibility.

2. **Releases Tension**: Alleviates tension and stiffness in the shoulders, neck, and upper back.
3. **Improves Circulation**: Encourages blood flow to the upper body, supporting muscle health and recovery.
4. **Strengthens Upper Body**: Engages the muscles of the arms and shoulders, contributing to upper body strength.
5. **Enhances Coordination and Motor Skills**: The rhythmic movement improves coordination and control of the arms and shoulders.

Instructions:
- Sit with feet flat on the floor.
- Extend arms out to the sides at shoulder height.
- Make small circles with your arms and gradually increase the size.
- Reverse the direction after several circles.

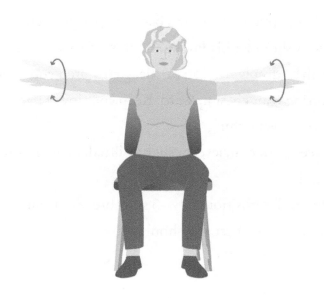

U3 Chair Cactus Arms with Back Arch

Benefits:

1. **Strengthens the upper back** and shoulder stabilizers.
2. **Encourages better posture** and spinal alignment.
3. **Reduces tension** in the neck and upper shoulders.
4. **Promotes circulation** and energy through the upper body.

Instructions:

- Sit tall in a sturdy chair with your feet flat on the floor and your spine upright.
- Lift your arms to shoulder height and bend your elbows to 90°, forming a "goalpost" or "cactus" shape. Spread your fingers wide.

- Gently pull your elbows back to open your chest, engaging your shoulder blades slightly toward each other.
- Inhale deeply. As you exhale, gently arch your upper back, lifting your chest upward. Keep your lower back stable and avoid overarching.
- Keep your chin level or slightly lifted, maintaining a relaxed neck.
- Hold this position for 2–3 slow breaths, feeling the stretch across your chest and shoulders.

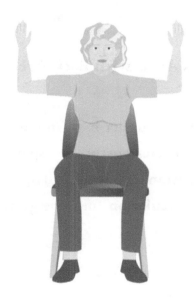

- On an exhale, bring your arms to the center, touching elbows and hands together in front of you.
- Repeat the opening and closing motion 5–10 times, moving with your breath.

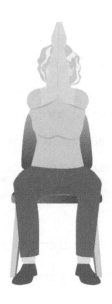

- To finish, lower your arms, return to a neutral spine, and relax your shoulders.

U4. Seated Shoulder Presses

This pose focuses on strengthening the shoulder muscles, particularly the deltoids, and improve upper body stability, posture, and arm mobility.

Benefits:
1. **Builds shoulder strength** and endurance.
2. **Enhances postural alignment** and shoulder stability.
3. **Engages the core** and upper back for better balance.
4. **Adaptable** for various fitness levels (can be done with or without weights).

59

Instructions:

- Sit tall in a sturdy chair with your feet flat on the floor, hip-width apart.
- Hold light dumbbells in each hand, elbows bent at 90°, palms facing forward, upper arms in line with your shoulders (goalpost position).
- Brace your core gently and keep your spine upright. Relax your shoulders away from your ears.
- Inhale to prepare. Exhale as you slowly press your arms upward until your elbows are almost straight—avoid locking them. Keep your movements controlled.
- Inhale as you lower your arms back to the starting position with control.

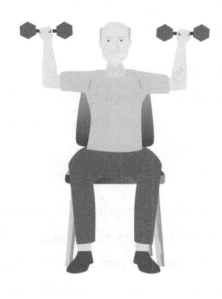

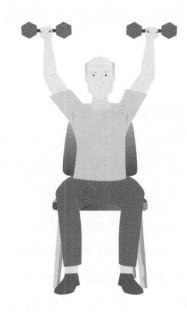

- Perform 8–12 reps, 1–3 sets, depending on your strength and comfort level.

- Move steadily, avoiding jerking or using momentum.

Modifications:

- Use no weights or household items like water bottles if dumbbells aren't available.

- Keep the range of motion smaller if you feel any shoulder discomfort.

Chapter 6 - Stretching & Relaxation Poses

S1. Seated Neck Stretches

These stretches focus on releasing tension and improving flexibility in the neck, shoulders, and upper back.

Instructions:

- Sit upright on a chair with feet flat on the floor. Relax your shoulders and keep your back straight.
- Neck Tilt: Gently tilt your head to the right, bringing your ear toward your right shoulder. Hold for 15-30 seconds, feeling the stretch on the left side of your neck.
- Return to center, tilt your head to the left, bringing your ear toward your left shoulder. Hold for 15-30 seconds.
- Return to center. Drop your chin toward your chest, stretching the back of your neck. Hold for 15-30 seconds.
- Gently tilt your head back, stretching the front of your neck. Hold for 10-15 seconds.
- Shoulder Support (Optional): Place your right hand on the left side of your head while tilting for a deeper stretch. Place your left hand on the right side of your head while tilting.
- Lateral Rotation (Optional): Slowly turn your head to the right, looking over your shoulder. Hold for 15-30 seconds, then switch sides.

- Finish by returning to a neutral position; breathe deeply throughout.

Precautions:

- Perform stretches gently, avoiding sudden movements.

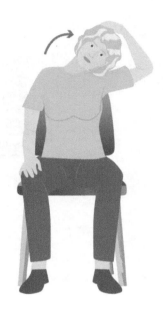

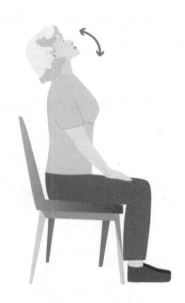

S2. Seated Shoulder Rolls

This pose focuses on improving mobility and relieving tension in the shoulder and neck area.

Instructions:

- Sit with your hands resting on your knees.
- Slowly roll your shoulders forward and up, then back and down.
- Repeat several times, then reverse the direction.

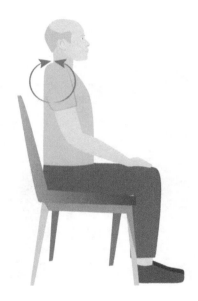

S3. Seated Cat-Cow Stretch

This combo pose focuses on enhancing spinal flexibility and promoting fluid movement through the back.

Instructions:

- Sit with feet flat on the floor.
- Inhale, arch your back and look slightly upwards (Cow Pose).
- Exhale, round your back, and tuck your chin to your chest (Cat Pose).
- Alternate between Cat and Cow with each breath for a few cycles.

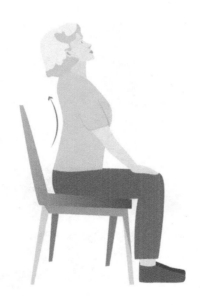

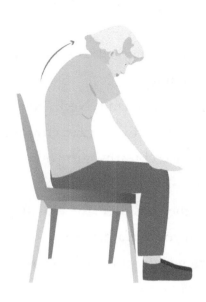

S4. Seated Chest Opener

This pose focuses on stretching and opening the chest, shoulders, and upper back. It counters the effects of poor posture, such as slouching or rounded shoulders.

Instructions:

- Sit on a sturdy chair with your feet flat on the floor, hip-width apart. Sit up tall with your back straight and shoulders relaxed.
- Reach your arms behind you and interlace your fingers. If interlacing is difficult, hold onto the edges of the chair or use a strap or towel between your hands.
- Open the Chest: Straighten your arms and gently pull them back, lifting your chest toward the ceiling. Draw your

shoulder blades together and down your back to enhance the stretch.

- Keep your core engaged to protect your lower back and avoid overarching.
- Adjust Your Head and Neck. Keep your chin slightly tucked or gently lift your gaze, ensuring no neck strain.
- Take slow, deep breaths into your chest, expanding your lungs fully.
- Maintain the position for 20-30 seconds or longer, focusing on your breath.
- Slowly bring your arms back to your sides and return to a neutral seated position.

Precautions:

This simple stretch is highly effective for improving posture, releasing tension, and revitalizing energy. However, don't overextend your body, consider the following tips.

- Avoid hunching your shoulders; keep them relaxed and down.
- If your lower back feels strained, sit further back on the chair for support.
- Perform the pose gently, ensuring no discomfort in your shoulders or chest.

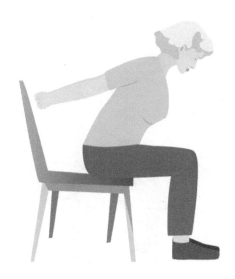

S5. Seated Side Stretch

This pose focuses on stretching the sides of the body, primarily targeting the obliques and intercostal muscles along the ribs.

Instructions:

- Sit tall on a chair with feet flat on the floor, hip-width apart.
- Rest your left hand on the chair seat or your left thigh.
- Inhale and extend your right arm overhead.
- Exhale as you lean your upper body to the left, keeping your right arm extended and your gaze towards the ceiling or straight ahead.
- Feel the stretch along the right side of your body.
- Hold for a few breaths, then return to the starting position.
- Repeat on the other side.

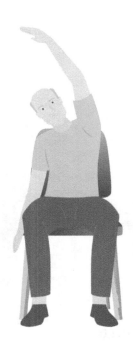

S6. Seated Spinal Twist

This pose focuses on stretching the back and hamstrings while promoting relaxation.

Instructions:

- Sit sideways on the chair with your right side facing the backrest.
- Place your right hand on the back of the chair.
- Inhale, lengthen your spine; exhale, gently twist to the right.
- Hold for a few breaths, then switch sides.
- Sit sideways on the chair with your left side facing the backrest.

- Place your left hand on the back of the chair.
- Inhale, lengthen your spine; exhale, gently twist to the left.
- Hold for a few breaths, then return to the forward-facing position.

Precautions:
- Gradually increase how far you can twist your upper body.
- Hold your breaths for the duration that you are comfortable with.

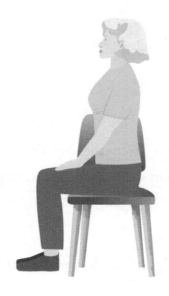

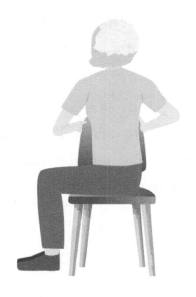

S7. Chair Pigeon

This pose focuses on strengthening the legs and lower body, enhancing flexibility in the hip joints, and improving balance and coordination.

Instructions:

- Sit near the edge of the chair with your feet flat on the floor, hip-width apart.
- Sit up tall with your back straight and shoulders relaxed. Keep your spine neutral and engage your core for stability.
- Lift your right leg and place your right ankle on your left thigh, just above the knee. Flex your right foot to protect the knee joint.

- Let your right knee drop naturally toward the floor, creating a figure-four shape. Ensure there's no strain or discomfort in the lifted knee.
- Gently press your right knee downward using your hand (optional) for a deeper stretch. Lean slightly forward from your hips, keeping your back straight. Avoid rounding your spine; lead with your chest as you fold forward.
- Hold the position for 20-30 seconds or longer, breathing deeply. Feel the stretch in your hips, glutes, and lower back.
- Slowly return to an upright position and lower your right leg to the floor.
- Repeat the pose with your left leg on top of your right thigh.

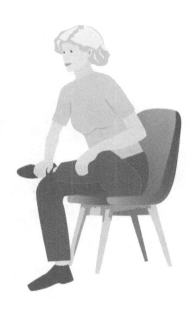

S8. Ankle Rolls

This pose focuses on improving mobility and flexibility in the ankle joints.

Instructions:

- Sit comfortably with your feet off the floor.
- Lift one foot or put one foot on the other knee and begin to roll the ankle clockwise, then counterclockwise.
- Switch to the other foot and repeat.

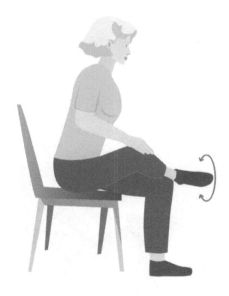

S9. Toe Taps

This combo pose focuses on improving mobility and circulation in the feet and lower legs.

Instructions:

- Sit with feet flat on the floor.
- Lift toes off the floor, keeping heels down, then lower toes back down.
- Lift heels off the floor, keeping the toes on the floor, then lower heels back down.
- Repeat several times.

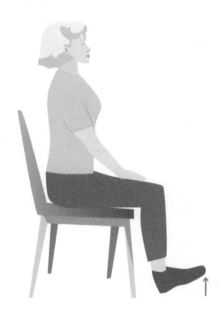

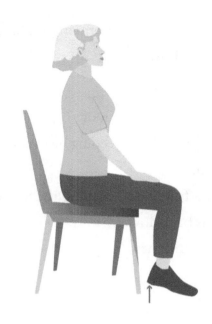

S10. Seated Relaxation

This is usually the final pose of your daily routine. It promotes calmness, relaxation, and mindfulness.

Instructions:

- Sit back comfortably with feet flat on the floor.
- Rest hands on thighs or lap.
- Close your eyes, take slow, deep breaths, inhale, hold for 5 seconds, and exhale. Relax your body completely.
- Stay in this pose and repeat deep breathing for 60 seconds or longer. Let go of any tension. If random thoughts pop up, which is perfectly normal, simply acknowledge them, then focus on your breaths.

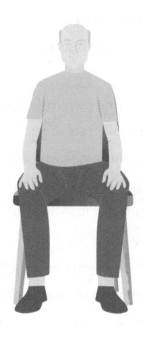

Chapter 7: 14-Day Challenge

Congratulations! You've learned 22 poses that focus on weight loss while increasing your overall mobility, flexibility, and energy. Now it's time to put them into action, incorporating them into a 10-minute daily routine. You don't need to do all 22 poses daily. I recommend purposely mixing a subset of them to target different parts of the body and help increase your metabolism for weight management or weight loss.

A 2021 study published in *Science* found that the metabolic rate begins to decrease by about 0.7 percent each year after age 60. This natural decline in metabolism can make it harder to maintain or lose weight as we age, contributing to weight gain and various health issues.

Consistently doing the same exercise without variation can lead to a plateau in your metabolic rate. Your body adapts to repetitive movements, becoming more efficient and burning fewer calories during each workout. As a result, you may hit a "plateau," where progress in calorie burning or muscle gain slows down, and you see minimal results.

Therefore, we want to work smarter, not harder, by mixing these poses. We'll change the routine after 7 days. This way, the 7-day repetitions help you master these poses, and changing the routine the following 7 days tricks the body into burning more calories. The routines are designed to progress in rigor. I intentionally did not assign duration for each pose to make it flexible during the learning phase. You're welcome to do more repetitions of a particular pose. Each pose plays a role, so try to follow the sequence in its entirety each time to maximize the benefits. Once you master these poses, you can easily finish each routine in 10 minutes or create your sequence of poses that could be 10 minutes long or longer.

Different theories exist regarding the number of consecutive days required to form a new long-term habit. Since I designed this guide to make chair yoga easy to do, help you immediately experience its benefits, and ensure you have fun, I trust you'll be motivated to practice the chair yoga poses in this book by the end of 14 days (2 weeks) or sooner.

To make things easier, I've included the number, name, instructions, and illustrations for each pose within every routine. This way, you can stay focused on your exercises without having to flip back and forth through pages. Each daily weight loss routine consists of 13 poses, ending with a relaxation pose. For Week 1, you'll repeat the same routine for 7 consecutive days to help you master the poses. In Week 2, you'll follow a different routine, also repeated for 7 days. Once you're familiar with the poses, feel free to mix and match them into your own 10-minute or longer routines. You're also welcome to use any of the stretching and relaxation poses in Chapter 6 throughout the day. The 13 poses in each daily routine are required during the 14-Day Challenge.

Week 1

Repeat this first routine of our 14-Day Challenge daily from Monday through Sunday during Week 1.

F1. Seated Mountain

- Sit up straight with feet flat on the floor, hip-width apart.
- Root your feet into the ground.
- Root your sitting bones into the chair.
- Lengthen your head toward the ceiling to create a neutral spine, engage your core, and lengthen your spine, imagining a string pulling the top of your head upwards.
- Extend your arms up, away from your ears, with your palms together.
- Keep your fingers soft and pointed up.
- Hold the pose for a few breaths.
- Drop your arms and relax your shoulders.

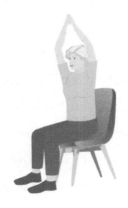

F2. Seated Warrior 1

- Sit sideways near the edge of the chair with feet flat on the floor, facing right.

- Extend your left leg back with toes on the floor; bend the front knee.

- Raise your arms upwards or leave your hands on your lap if needed.

- Hold for a few breaths, then switch sides.

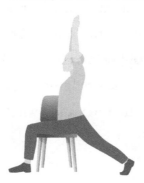

F3. Seated Warrior 2

- Sit sideways on a sturdy chair with your right side aligned with the chair's backrest. Ensure your right thigh is parallel to the chair seat and your feet are firmly planted on the ground.

- Extend your left leg to the side, keeping it straight, while your right leg remains bent at a 90-degree angle. Make sure both feet are flat on the ground, with the right foot facing forward and the left foot slightly turned. If keeping your left foot fully flat is uncomfortable, press firmly into the ball of your foot for stability.

- Stretch your arms out to the sides parallel to the floor, aligning them with your shoulders. Your fingertips should be active, extending in opposite directions.
- Keep your torso upright, facing toward the bent right knee. Engage your core to maintain balance and stability.
- Turn your head to gaze over your right fingertips, maintaining a relaxed neck and shoulders.
- Hold this position for several breaths, focusing on the stretch and engaging your muscles. Feel the stretch in your inner thighs and the strengthening of your core and arms.
- Gently release the pose and switch sides, repeating with your left knee bent.

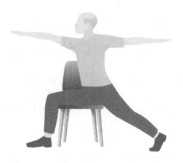

F4. Chair Crescent Lunge

- Sit sideways on the chair. Position your right hip facing the chair's backrest. Keep both feet flat on the floor.

- Slide the right leg back. Extend your right leg behind you. Keep the toes tucked under or flat on the floor, depending on your flexibility. Your left knee stays bent at 90°, directly over the left ankle.
- Square your hips forward as much as possible. Lengthen the spine. Sit tall and avoid arching your back.
- Reach your arms upward with palms facing each other. Keep your shoulders relaxed and down.

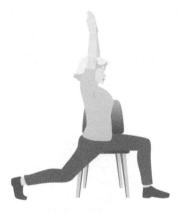

- Engage the core. Pull your navel toward the spine. Stay in this position for 3–5 slow breaths.
- Turn your torso to face the chair's backrest. Extend your arms outward and hold for 2-3 slow breaths.

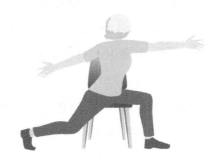

- Turn your torso, facing forward. Place your hands together in front of your chest, while keeping the right leg extended. Hold in this position for 2-3 slow breaths.

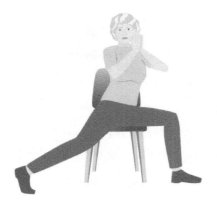

F5. Seated Jumping Jacks
- Sit tall in a sturdy chair. Keep your feet flat on the floor and core lightly engaged.
- Sit toward the front edge of the chair, keeping your spine long.

- Place your arms at your sides and feet together.

- Raise your arms overhead in a wide "V" shape. At the same time, step your feet out wide to the sides.

- Lower your arms back to your sides and step your feet back together.

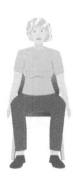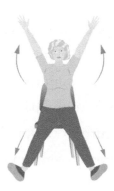

- Repeat at a steady rhythm. Aim for 8–12 repetitions, or continue for 30–60 seconds at a gentle pace

- Breathe naturally and move within your comfort range.

C1. Seated Hip Circles

- Sit on a sturdy chair with your feet flat on the floor, hip-width apart. Sit upright with your back straight and shoulders relaxed.

- Engage your abdominal muscles to support your lower back during the movement.

- Slowly shift your torso forward, moving in a circular motion to the right.

- Lean your torso to the right, then circle it back, rounding through the lower back.
- Continue the circle to the left and return to the starting position.
- Keep the movement slow and smooth, creating a rhythmic flow.
- Repeat: Complete 5-10 circles in one direction, then reverse the direction for an equal number of circles.
- Breathe mindfully. Inhale as you circle forward and exhale as you round back.
- Return to an upright position and take a few deep breaths before moving on.

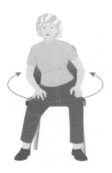

C2. Seated Torso Twist

- Sit tall with feet flat on the floor, hip-width apart.
- Place your left hand on the right knee and your right hand on the back of the chair.
- Inhale to lengthen the spine, exhale to twist your torso to the right gently.
- Hold for a few breaths, then repeat on the other side.

For a more advanced version, place your left hand on the right edge of your seat, your right hand on the back of the chair, and turn your upper body and neck more. Repeat the same on the other side. You should feel your core tightening as you twist.

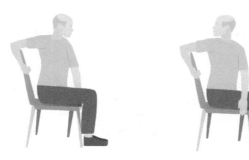

C3. Chair Boat Pose

- Sit closer to the edge of the chair with your knees bent and feet flat.
- Lean back slightly, keeping your back straight.
- Lift your feet off the floor, balancing on your sit bones.
- Keep your arms parallel to the floor or hold the sides of the chair for support.
- Hold for a few breaths, then lower your feet.

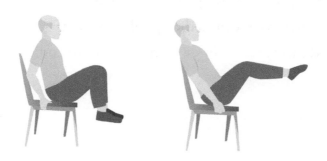

C4. Seated Forward Bend

- Sit tall with feet flat on the floor.
- Inhale, lengthen your spine.
- Exhale, hinge at the hips, and lean forward, reaching your hands towards your feet.
- Hold gently for a few deep breaths, then slowly rise back.

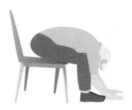

C5. Chair Side Bend

- Sit straight on a chair with both feet flat on the ground, hip-width apart.
- Place your right hand behind your head and your left hand on your hip or down by your side.
- Inhale to prepare; as you exhale, bend your torso to the left, bringing your right elbow towards your left side.
- Keep your chest open and core engaged.
- Inhale to return to the upright position.
- Repeat several times, then switch to the other side.

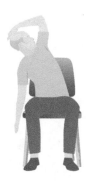

C6. Seated Marching

- Sit tall with feet flat on the floor.
- Alternate lifting each knee towards your chest as if marching.
- Keep your core engaged throughout the movement.
- Increase the speed gradually for a cardiovascular effect.

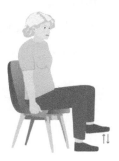

L1. Seated Knee Lifts

- Sit tall with feet flat on the floor.
- Lift one knee towards your chest, engaging your core.
- Hold for a moment, then lower it back down.
- Alternate legs, performing the movement in a controlled manner.

- The longer you hold, the more you're exercising your core muscles. Be sure to breathe in and out.

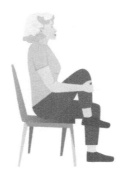

L4. Chair Tree

- Sit tall, keep your feet flat and spine straight.
- Place your right foot on your left knee.
- Engage your core, and focus on a point ahead.
- Hands in prayer at the chest or overhead.
- Maintain for several breaths, then switch sides.

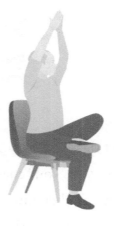

S10. Seated Relaxation

- Sit back comfortably with feet flat on the floor.

- Rest hands on thighs or lap.
- Close your eyes, take slow, deep breaths, inhale, hold for 5 seconds, and exhale. Relax your body completely.
- Stay in this pose and repeat deep breathing for 60 seconds or longer. Let go of any tension. If random thoughts pop up, which is perfectly normal, simply acknowledge them, then focus on your breaths.

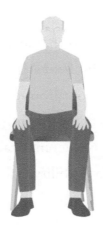

Week 2

Repeat this first routine of our 14-Day Challenge daily from Monday through Sunday during Week 2.

F3. Seated Warrior 2

- Sit sideways on a sturdy chair with your right side aligned with the chair's backrest. Ensure your right thigh is parallel to the chair seat and your feet are firmly planted on the ground.
- Extend your left leg to the side, keeping it straight, while your right leg remains bent at a 90-degree angle. Make sure both feet are flat on the ground, with the right foot facing forward and the left foot slightly turned. If keeping your left foot fully flat is uncomfortable, press firmly into the ball of your foot for stability.

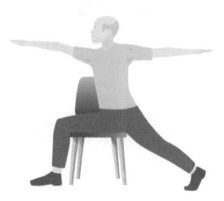

- Stretch your arms out to the sides parallel to the floor, aligning them with your shoulders. Your fingertips should be active, extending in opposite directions.

- Keep your torso upright, facing toward the bent right knee. Engage your core to maintain balance and stability.

- Turn your head to gaze over your right fingertips, maintaining a relaxed neck and shoulders.

- Hold this position for several breaths, focusing on the stretch and engaging your muscles. Feel the stretch in your inner thighs and the strengthening of your core and arms.

- Gently release the pose and switch sides, repeating with your left knee bent.

F5. Seated Jumping Jacks

- Sit tall in a sturdy chair. Keep your feet flat on the floor and core lightly engaged.

- Sit toward the front edge of the chair, keeping your spine long.

- Place your arms at your sides and feet together.

- Raise your arms overhead in a wide "V" shape. At the same time, step your feet out wide to the sides.

- Lower your arms back to your sides and step your feet back together.

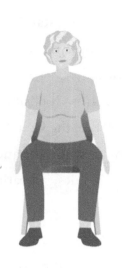
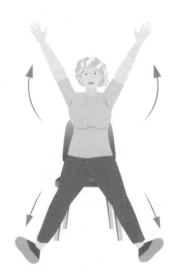

F6. Seated Kick Punches

- Lift your right leg off the floor.

- At the same time, punch your left arm across your body (diagonally toward the right)

- Keep your back straight — don't lean.

- Return to start — Gently lower your leg and arm back to the starting position.

- Breathe naturally — exhale as you punch/kick, inhale as you return. Start slow and build a steady rhythm.

- Switch sides — Lift your left leg and punch your right arm forward

- Keep alternating sides: **right kick + left punch, then left kick + right punch**.

94

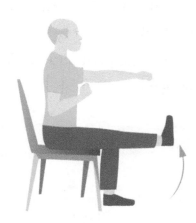

C1. Seated Hip Circles

- Sit on a sturdy chair with your feet flat on the floor, hip-width apart. Sit upright with your back straight and shoulders relaxed.
- Engage your abdominal muscles to support your lower back during the movement. Slowly shift your torso forward, moving in a circular motion to the right.
- Lean your torso to the right, then circle it back, rounding through the lower back.
- Continue the circle to the left and return to the starting position.
- Keep the movement slow and smooth, creating a rhythmic flow.
- Repeat: Complete 5-10 circles in one direction, then reverse the direction for an equal number of circles.

- Breathe mindfully. Inhale as you circle forward and exhale as you round back.
- Return to an upright position and take a few deep breaths before moving on.

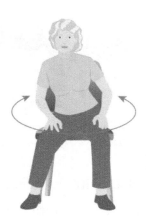

C5. Chair Side Bend

- Sit straight on a chair with both feet flat on the ground, hip-width apart.
- Place your right hand behind your head and your left hand on your hip or down by your side.
- Inhale to prepare; as you exhale, bend your torso to the left, bringing your right elbow towards your left side.
- Keep your chest open and core engaged.
- Inhale to return to the upright position.
- Repeat for several repetitions, then switch to the other side.

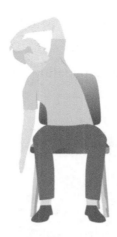

C6. Seated Marching

- Sit tall with feet flat on the floor.
- Alternate lifting each knee towards your chest as if marching.
- Keep your core engaged throughout the movement.
- Increase the speed gradually for a cardiovascular effect.

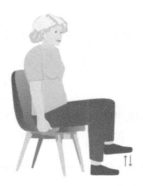

C7. Seated Bicycle Crunches

- Sit near the edge of a sturdy chair with feet flat on the floor.
- Lightly place your hands behind your head.

- Bring your right elbow towards your left knee while extending your right leg.
- Alternate sides in a pedaling motion, keeping the core engaged.

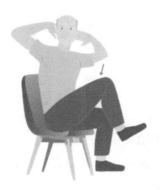

U1. Seated Eagle Arms

- Sit with feet flat on the floor.
- Cross your right arm under the left, wrapping at the elbows.
- Try to bring palms together or as close as possible.
- Lift elbows slightly and hold for a few breaths, then switch arms.
- Cross your left arm under the right, wrapping at the elbows.
- Try to bring palms together or as close as possible.
- Lift elbows slightly and hold for a few breaths.

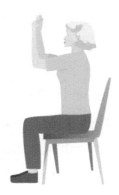

U2. Seated Arm Circles

- Sit with feet flat on the floor.
- Extend arms out to the sides at shoulder height.
- Make small circles with your arms and gradually increase the size.
- Reverse the direction after several circles.

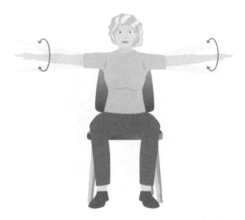

U3 Chair Cactus Arms with Back Arch

- Sit tall in a sturdy chair with your feet flat on the floor and your spine upright.

- Lift your arms to shoulder height and bend your elbows to 90°, forming a "goalpost" or "cactus" shape. Spread your fingers wide.
- Gently pull your elbows back to open your chest, engaging your shoulder blades slightly toward each other.
- Inhale deeply. As you exhale, gently arch your upper back, lifting your chest upward. Keep your lower back stable and avoid overarching.
- Keep your chin level or slightly lifted, maintaining a relaxed neck.
- Hold this position for 2–3 slow breaths, feeling the stretch across your chest and shoulders.

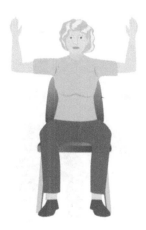

- On an exhale, bring your arms to the center, touching elbows and hands together in front of you.
- Repeat the opening and closing motion 5–10 times, moving with your breath.

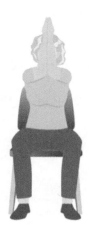

U4. Seated Shoulder Presses

- Sit tall in a sturdy chair with your feet flat on the floor, hip-width apart.
- Hold light dumbbells (or water bottles) in each hand, elbows bent at 90°, palms facing forward, upper arms in line with your shoulders (goalpost position).
- Brace your core gently and keep your spine upright. Relax your shoulders away from your ears.

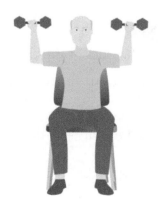

- Inhale to prepare. Exhale as you slowly press your arms upward until your elbows are almost straight—avoid locking them. Keep your movements controlled.

- Inhale as you lower your arms back to the starting position with control.

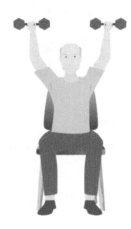

- Perform 8–12 reps, 1–3 sets, depending on your strength and comfort level.

- Move steadily, avoiding jerking or using momentum.

L2. Seated Leg Lifts
- Sit tall and grip the sides of the chair.
- Lift one leg straight out in front of you and hold for 3-4 slow breaths.
- Lower the leg and repeat with the other leg.

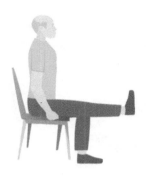

L3. Seated Hamstring Stretch with Core Hold

- Sit upright on a sturdy chair, feet flat on the floor, spine tall.
- Extend one leg forward, straightening the knee as much as possible, heel resting on the floor with toes pointing up.
- Engage the core by gently drawing the navel toward the spine.
- Place hands on the opposite thigh or rest gently on the sides of the extended leg (avoid pushing on the knee).
- Hinge forward slightly from the hips, keeping the back flat and long. Avoid rounding the spine.
- Hold this stretch while keeping the core engaged. Breathe slowly and steadily.
- Stay in this position for 3–5 deep breaths. Feel the stretch in the back of the extended leg while maintaining a stable, active core.

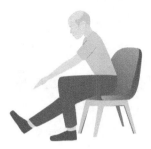

- Return to upright, bend the extended leg, and place the foot flat.
- Repeat on the other side.

S10. Seated Relaxation

- Sit back comfortably with feet flat on the floor.
- Rest hands on thighs or lap.
- Close your eyes, take slow, deep breaths, inhale, hold for 5 seconds, and exhale. Relax your body completely.
- Stay in this pose and repeat deep breathing for 60 seconds or longer. Let go of any tension. If random thoughts pop up, which is perfectly normal, simply acknowledge them, then focus on your breaths.

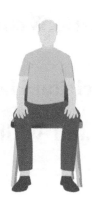

Bonus Holistic Wellness Guide

Chapter 8: Nutrition Hacks for Weight Loss and Wellness

Have you heard the saying, "We are what we eat?" Although it's not literal, it does imply that the food we consume has a significant impact on our overall physical and mental health.

If you often feel tired and lethargic, inadequate nutrition could be the problem. You keep gaining weight while eating the same amount of food when you were younger. Nourishing your body with quality nutrients can positively impact your physical and mental well-being. Many nutrition and diet books are available so that we won't delve into detailed nutrition information. However, making smart nutrition choices is the key to fueling your body and managing your weight.

Sustained fat loss requires a true calorie deficit meaning you burn more calories than you consume; however, individual results may vary due to factors such as metabolism, hormones, and the accuracy of tracking. Starving oneself never works. Intermittent fasting works for some people, but it is not easy for all to get used to. Therefore, I will share several key nutrition hacks backed by science and real-life success stories from my Amazon Best Seller –

Weight Loss Hacks for Women Over 40, to make your weight loss journey enjoyable.

Boost Energy While Limiting Calories

Lower-nutrient, high-calorie foods can quickly cause your blood sugar to spike, leaving you feeling lethargic. Smart nutrition choices include replacing these with higher nutrients and lower-calorie foods. These foods will fuel and nourish your body, helping you feel full and stay energized while managing your calorie consumption and weight.

Seniors need to eat high-protein foods to help maintain muscle mass and strength, which can decline with age. To fuel your body in the morning and throughout the day, consider consuming foods that energize your body with essential nutrients, including protein, unsaturated fats, fiber, minerals, and vitamins. Smart nutrition choices include lean proteins, nuts and seeds, nut butter, whole grains, leafy greens, and fruits such as avocados, tomatoes, and oranges, which have lower sugar content but are rich in nutrients.

Prediabetes Can Be Reversed

According to a survey, the prevalence of diabetes and prediabetes among people aged 40–49 is 11.1% and 40.3%, respectively. The good news is prediabetes can be reversed through proper nutrition and weight management, such as reducing the intake of refined carbs (e.g., white rice, white bread, white pasta, etc.), added sugars (e.g., sugary beverages, cookies, cakes, candy, etc.), saturated and trans fats (e.g., butter, sausages, bacon, cheese, etc.).

Limit Foods That Cause Inflammation & Weight Gain

Foods high in saturated fats, refined grains, and added sugars can cause inflammation and weight gain. These include:

Red Meat: Steak, hamburgers, and other red meat products

Processed Meats: Bacon, sausage, bologna, lunch meat, and hot dogs

Refined Grains: White bread, white rice, pasta, and breakfast cereals

Fried Foods: French fries, fried chicken, and donuts

Commercial Baked Goods: Cookies, pies, brownies, and snack cakes

Added Sugars: Candy, cookies, soda, bread, crackers, granola bars, salad dressings, yogurt, and cereals

Trans Fats: These fats, found in packaged foods, raise bad cholesterol without increasing good cholesterol

Some of you might be frustrated after seeing this list. It sounds like you can't eat many of your favorite foods. For some individuals, reducing their carbohydrate intake can be a challenge. You can substitute refined grains with healthy carbs (whole grains) and fiber-rich foods to help you feel full. Refine grains are low in nutrients and high in calories.

The instant gratification of feeling full from eating bread and pasta is temporary. Eating refined grains can cause blood sugar to spike and then crash because they are digested quickly and have little nutritional value. And you will feel hungry not long after.

Doing anything extreme is not sustainable. The best way to interpret this list is to reduce intake or find substitutes rather than eliminating these foods. If you can start by minimizing processed meats and reducing added sugar, you are already making significant progress in making smart choices.

Train Your Taste Buds and Control Sugar, Sodium, and Fat Intake

Our taste buds are capable of evolving. You can enjoy foods with 25% less sugar, sodium, or butter in just a few weeks by gradually reducing intake and training your taste buds to appreciate less sugar, sodium, and fat in your diet.

If you are retired, consider cooking more meals instead of grabbing snacks from pre-packaged bags that often contain high levels of sodium or sugar. Instead of buying muffins and cakes from the store, bake your desserts at home, where you can gradually reduce the amount of sugar, butter, and oil you use.

If you use soy sauce to stir-fry or marinate meat, opt for soy sauce with a lower sodium content. In about 3-4 weeks, you will get used to the flavor. Similarly, you can gradually reduce the amount of salt and butter you use for cooking; that way, you won't feel the food is too bland, and you will be more motivated to control your sugar, sodium, and overall fat intake.

When you go out to eat, you can ask your server to request that your order be prepared with less oil or salt in freshly cooked foods. Some sauces are pre-made. Then, you ask the server to put pre-made sauces on the side, so you get to control how much you put on your dish.

Hacks to Control Cravings

Why do we often consume more calories than the body really needs? It could be caused by stress, low blood sugar levels, a lack of quality nutrients, or confusing hunger with another sensation, such as dehydration. The following super simple hacks are not new inventions; however, I'm going to make it easy for you to incorporate them into your daily life so that you can turn these mini habits into lifelong routines for sustainable weight loss.

Cravings Control Hack #1 – Warm Water

Because some of the symptoms of dehydration can resemble symptoms of hunger (e.g., fatigue, lightheadedness), let's ensure your body does not confuse thirst with hunger, which can cause you to overeat.

When you first wake up, drink warm water, preferably not cold water, coffee, or juice. Drinking warm water can kick-start your metabolism. Keeping yourself hydrated can help prevent your brain from confusing dehydration with hunger; therefore, you will be less tempted to grab high-calorie foods such as donuts or bagels in front of you.

Cravings Control Hack #2a – Apple Cider Vinegar

Vinegar has many health benefits, including supporting weight loss. Taking vinegar directly is torture, but you can take apple cider vinegar capsules as an alternative. That way, you cannot taste anything sour. Apple cider vinegar contains acetic acid, which is known to reduce the absorption of carbohydrates, can help the body burn more fat, and may provide a feeling of fullness.

You can easily find apple cider vinegar capsules on Amazon. Make sure to read the reviews and consider purchasing brands with a high number of reviews and an average rating of 4.3 stars or higher.

Cravings Control Hack #2b – Warm Lemon Water

If you prefer drinking acidic water, you can try fresh lemon water as an alternative. There are scientific studies on the benefits of drinking lemon water in the morning, including boosting energy and alertness, as well as increasing bowel movements.

You can simply hand-squeeze half of a lemon into a glass of warm water. Depending on where you live, the cost of a bottle of apple cider vinegar capsules that typically lasts 30 days might be similar to the cost of buying fresh lemons. You don't have to consume a full glass of warm lemon water at once in the morning. You can add lemon to your mid-morning or afternoon tea.

Cravings Control Hack #3 – Nut Butter

When it comes to managing cravings and maintaining a balanced diet, nut butter is an unexpected yet effective ally. At first glance, it might seem counterintuitive to consume fats when trying to lose body fat. However, incorporating healthy fats, such as those found in nut butter, can play a crucial role in achieving your wellness goals.

Nut butter, including almond, peanut, and cashew butter, is rich in monounsaturated and polyunsaturated fats. These healthy fats promote satiety, meaning they help you feel full for more extended periods. By satisfying hunger more effectively, nut butter can reduce the likelihood of reaching for unhealthy snacks between meals.

Additionally, nut butter is packed with protein and fiber, which further enhances its satiating effect. This powerful combination helps stabilize blood sugar levels, preventing the spikes and crashes that often lead to cravings for sugary or high-carb treats.

Incorporating moderate amounts of nut butter into your diet can also provide essential nutrients, including vitamin E, magnesium, and antioxidants. These nutrients support overall health and wellness, complementing your weight loss efforts.

To make the most of this cravings control hack, enjoy nut butter as a spread on whole-grain toast, blend it into smoothies, or use it as a dip for fresh fruits and vegetables. Just remember to choose natural, unsweetened varieties to avoid added sugars and unhealthy fats. By embracing the benefits of nut butter, you can satisfy your cravings the healthy way and advance your journey toward weight loss and overall wellness.

Cravings Control Hack #4 – Leafy Greens

Incorporating leafy green salads into your daily routine can be a game-changer when it comes to managing cravings and supporting your wellness journey. Leafy greens, such as spinach, kale, arugula, and romaine lettuce, are nutritional powerhouses that offer numerous benefits for those seeking weight loss and overall health.

One of the standout features of leafy greens is their high fiber content. Fiber plays a vital role in promoting satiety, helping you feel full sooner and stay satisfied for a more extended period. By curbing hunger pangs and reducing the temptation to snack on less healthy options, leafy greens can help effectively control cravings.

In addition to fiber, leafy greens are loaded with essential vitamins and minerals that our bodies need for optimal functioning. They provide a rich source of vitamins A, C, K, and several B vitamins, as well as minerals such as calcium, potassium, and magnesium. These nutrients contribute to enhanced energy levels, immune system support, and overall well-being.

Leafy greens also contribute to the body's natural detoxification processes. Chlorophyll, found abundantly in greens, aids in eliminating toxins and promoting liver health. This detoxifying effect not only supports weight management but also boosts your sense of well-being.

Leafy Green Salads With Lean Proteins & Nuts

To make leafy green salads both easy and enjoyable, consider experimenting with a variety of greens and toppings. Incorporate colorful vegetables, nuts, seeds, or protein sources such as boiled eggs, grilled chicken, salmon, lean beef brisket, or tofu. Dressing your salad with a simple combination of olive oil and apple or lemon vinaigrette can provide a refreshing and nutritious flavor profile while avoiding the heaviness of cheese. This salad preparation can take as little as 2 minutes if the proteins are already done.

Lightly Boiled With Soups

It's not uncommon for some to compare eating leafy green salads to chewing grass, particularly with greens like arugula that have a distinct, peppery flavor. Arugula can be an acquired taste, but it can be quite enjoyable when prepared creatively. For instance, you can alternate between eating it raw or adding it to your bone broth soup just before serving. By letting it blanch quickly in the hot broth for a couple of minutes, the arugula softens while still retaining most of its nutrients, offering a delightful twist to your meal. You can do the same experiment with spinach.

Steam Greens for a Softer Texture

For those who find raw greens too fibrous or have a taste likened to "chewing grass," steaming offers a fantastic alternative. You can steam leafy greens like spinach, as well as other vegetables like green beans, bok choy, and broccoli, to achieve a softer texture while retaining their vibrant color and nutrients.

Steaming is a straightforward process that can be easily done at home with a pot and a steamer insert. Here's a simple method to steam your greens for a pleasant texture:

1. **Setup**: Fill a pot with 1 or 2 inches of water and bring it to a gentle boil.

2. **Steamer Insert**: Place a stainless steel steamer plate or basket inside the pot, ensuring it doesn't touch the water directly.

3. **Prepare Vegetables**: Wash your vegetables thoroughly and place them evenly on the steamer plate.

4. **Steaming**: Cover the pot with a lid and let the vegetables steam for 5 to 15 minutes, depending on the vegetable and desired level of softness.

5. **Finishing Touches**: Once steamed to your liking, carefully remove the vegetables and season them with salt or your favorite sauce for enhanced flavor.

This method not only softens the greens and vegetables, making them more palatable, but also helps retain their essential vitamins and minerals. You can add steamed greens to your salads for a warm variation or serve as a side dish, providing a delightful and nourishing element to your meal.

Cravings Control Hack #5 — Eat Low-Sugar Fruits, Nuts and Seeds as Snacks or Deserts

Incorporating low-sugar fruits, such as berries, watermelon, oranges, avocados, and tomatoes, into your diet is an excellent way to manage cravings.

Berries, including blueberries, raspberries, strawberries, and blackberries, are not only delicious but also rich in antioxidants and proanthocyanidins, which may help prevent and combat heart disease and cancer. They support brain health, aid digestion with their high fiber content, and provide immune support with vitamins C and K.

Watermelon is a hydrating and low-calorie treat, making it a refreshing choice for a sweet snack. It contains vitamins A and C and is rich in antioxidants, offering a natural way to satisfy your sweet tooth while supporting overall wellness. Enjoy these fruits fresh, blended in smoothies, or as a natural dessert alternative to enhance your diet with delicious and nutritious choices. Minimize or avoid drinking soda or fruit juices you get from stores that usually contain added sugar. Instead, eat watermelon or make smoothies at home by blending all-natural fruits only.

Avocados and tomatoes are also low-sugar and nutritious fruits. In culinary terms, both are often treated as vegetables due to their savory flavors. They also make excellent snacks.

Nuts and seeds are an incredibly nutritious addition to your snack and dessert rotation, offering a powerhouse of health benefits to complement your wellness goals. Rich in antioxidants, these tiny nutritional giants help combat oxidative stress in the body, protecting your cells and reducing the risk of chronic diseases. The high fiber content in nuts and seeds aids digestion, promotes a feeling of fullness, and helps manage cravings, making them an ideal choice for those seeking to manage their weight.

A Word on the "Pink Salt Trick" for Weight Loss

In recent years, Himalayan pink salt has gained popularity not only as a culinary staple but also as an ingredient in various health and wellness practices, including those aimed at weight loss. The "pink salt trick" involves integrating Himalayan pink salt into a balanced diet, with some believing it offers health benefits that may assist in weight management.

Himalayan pink salt is renowned for its unique mineral composition, boasting over **80 trace minerals**, including magnesium, calcium, and potassium. **These minerals contribute to improved hydration and electrolyte balance, which are crucial for sustaining energy levels and enhancing metabolic efficiency. Proper hydration, in turn, supports digestion and can help curb cravings, facilitating more effective calorie management.**

While pink salt itself lacks direct fat-burning properties, it enhances the flavor of healthy meals, providing a satisfying alternative to other high-sodium seasonings that may cause water retention. **Using pink salt in moderation can help avoid**

excessive sodium intake associated with processed table salt, which is often linked to bloating and impeded weight loss efforts.

For some, starting the day with a glass of warm water mixed with a pinch of pink salt and lemon is believed to invigorate metabolism, cleanse the body, and support digestive health — factors that can be beneficial in a weight loss journey. However, it's essential to approach the pink salt trick with realism and incorporate it as part of a balanced and nutritious overall diet. Relying solely on pink salt for weight loss is unlikely to yield significant results without the foundation of strategic nutritional practices, regular physical activity, and mindful lifestyle choices.

Despite its nuanced flavor profile, which tastes less salty than regular salt, excessive sodium consumption in any form remains unhealthy and can cause water retention. Adding a pinch of pink salt to a glass of warm lemon water or tea during the day, using it in cooking, and mixing a small amount into a glass of warm water in the evening is quite refreshing and more enjoyable.

In summary, while Himalayan pink salt can enhance your diet with its distinct flavor and mineral content, it should be regarded as a supportive element within a broader, comprehensive approach to health and weight management.

Next, I'd like to share another category of nature's gifts to support weight loss and enrich your wellness lifestyle.

Chapter 9: Herbal Support for Weight Loss and Wellness

It's tempting to try Ozempic, which got popularized as the magical weight loss medication, although it was initially designed for managing type 2 diabetes. Many users have also reported its side effects, including celebrities. Natural solutions such as herbal remedies, when taken in moderation, can also support weight loss without harmful side effects. Some people ended up staying in the hospital for months after taking what seemed to be regularly prescribed medications for treating common illnesses. The side effect of one drug can result in a domino effect to deteriorate one's health. I'm a firm believer in holistic wellness, leveraging nature's gifts while staying informed on scientific facts.

I'll share several highly accessible herb remedies that can support your weight loss journey. You may have already heard of these terms, HCA and EGCG, in weight loss supplement commercials. Guess what? You can gain access to these ingredients directly by sourcing the origin of these weight loss support ingredients at your local grocery store without spending a fortune on diet pills that may cause side effects.

Effective Herbs for Appetite Control and Fat Burning

Hibiscus

A tropical plant, hibiscus thrives in a humid and warm tropical climate. Unlike most medicinal plants used for tea, in this case, the flower is used—not leaves or bark. Hibiscus is an excellent, natural, and rich source of Hydroxycut or hydroxy citric acid (HCA), the key chemical in most diet formulas. It also contains chromium and ascorbic acid, two potent chemicals that help fight obesity.

Hibiscus is typically consumed as a tea (made from flowers), but in Mexico, hibiscus flowers are used to create a delicious and potent wine. The tea or wine is a rich source of Vitamin C and has light, laxative, and diuretic properties. You can try the tea flowers—hibiscus is easy to find in health food stores, shops, and online, usually sold as dried petals for making tart, refreshing tea. The calyx portion of the hibiscus flower is used for the tea after it is dried.

Garcinia Fruit

Garcinia is a native of India. It is used intensively in herbal medicinal formulas to treat bowel conditions and rheumatism. It is also prescribed as a heart tonic and to promote better digestion. This fruit is a rich source of HCA, which significantly enhances the metabolic rate, thereby aiding in weight loss.

The HCA extract from this fruit is extensively used in weight loss herbal formulas and is quite potent. It comes in capsule, tablet, and powder forms (for smoothies). Although you can consume the HCA extract as a tea, it is quite bitter. It is best to take it in capsules.

Some resources advise using whole fruit instead of tablets, capsules, or powders, as these do not contain potassium, which prevents the HCA from binding to calcium and, therefore, making it more difficult to absorb in the body. The fruit, on the other hand, can provide the required amounts of HCA without this downside.

Garcinia fruit can be found in local Whole Foods Markets or ethnic grocery stores that cater to customers from India and Southeast Asia. Suppose you can't easily purchase fresh garcinia fruit. In that case, you can buy it in capsule or powder form at local health and wellness stores, such as GNC, The Vitamin Shoppe, Whole Foods Market, or online retailers like Amazon.

Stevia

Stevia is a tropical plant that thrives in humid and warm climates. Though it can be grown from a seed, it is better to grow it as a sapling, as it will have a lower mortality rate. The leaves serve as natural sweeteners for individuals with diabetes or those seeking to avoid the drawbacks of refined sugar.

Stevia leaves and extracts are used primarily to treat diabetes by regulating blood sugar levels. Its use prevents the development of type 2 diabetes. It helps in weight loss by keeping the calorie count to a minimum (by eliminating sugar).

The sweet leaves of this plant are a pleasant and guilt-free alternative to sugar. However, when used fresh in teas, they leave a bitter aftertaste. Hence, the extract is preferred to its natural form, though some of its goodness is lost. Since it does not caramelize, it is not well-suited for baking sweets.

Stevia products are available at supermarkets like Walmart, Target, and Costco. These stores may sell powdered or liquid stevia under various brands. Specialty stores, such as Whole Foods Market, Trader Joe's, and Sprouts Farmers Market, are great places to find stevia in various forms.

Green Tea

Green tea is a great way to naturally lose body fat. Caffeine is a significant component of green tea, serving as a stimulant that helps you burn fat and enhances your ability to exercise more effectively. In a recent study, participants were given 4 to 5 cups of green tea daily for 12 weeks. These participants lost belly fat while simultaneously gaining muscle mass.

The most active ingredient in green tea is EGCG, which accounts for a significant portion of green tea's weight properties. EGCG not only helps boost your metabolism, allowing you to burn fat faster, but it also helps prevent your body from creating new fat cells. Your fat cells are responsible for weight gain; reducing their production makes gaining weight more difficult.

Green tea contains catechins, which help shrink belly fat. The catechins in green tea can aid your weight loss journey by helping to remove fat from fat cells, particularly those in the belly area.

According to a 2012 study, fourteen overweight individuals participated, losing an average of 0.2 to 3.5 kg in twelve weeks. This demonstrates the remarkable effectiveness of green tea in aiding natural weight loss without the risk of side effects or complications.

Green tea is universally available. You can find green teas in regional or nationwide chain stores as well as online retailers. There are different types of green tea. Try to obtain premium green tea types within your budget. To learn more about these simple herbal remedies, I highly recommend the book *Simplified Herbal Remedies for Beginners: Natural DIY Solutions for Immune Boost, Stress Relief, Insomnia, Pain Management, Heart Health, Gut Health, Weight Loss, and Lifelong Wellness.* by Aurora Hawthorne, available on Amazon.

You've just gained another tool to support your weight loss journey. Next, let's talk about losing weight through quality sleep.

Chapter 10: Sleep Your Way to Better Health and Weight Loss

Sleeping can help you lose weight, which may not sound intuitively obvious since a significant portion of the book focuses on staying active to lose weight.

One thing we can all agree on is that we cannot eat or drink while we sleep. So, sleeping more can reduce our calorie intake frequency and amount. It is common for older adults to experience changes in the quality and duration of their sleep. Many of these changes occur due to changes in the body's internal clock. This internal clock, known as the circadian rhythm, influences when we feel hungry, sleepy, or alert. As people age, the brain produces less melatonin, a hormone that plays a role in regulating sleep. Sleep homeostasis declines with age, leading to increased nighttime awakenings. Other factors that can impact sleep quality include medications and medical conditions. Insomnia, sleep apnea, and restless legs syndrome are common sleep disorders in older adults. Now that you have a new and fun daily chair yoga routine ensure you get quality sleep and stay alert when practicing chair yoga poses.

How Much Sleep Do You Need?

While sleep requirements vary from person to person, most healthy adults require seven to nine hours of sleep per night. The quality of sleep is more important than the quantity. Frequently waking up not feeling rested or tired during the day is the best indication that you're not getting enough sleep.

Proven Tips to Improve Sleep

- Avoid big meals or spicy foods before bed
- Reduce or avoid high-sodium foods that cause you to drink too much water before bed
- Limit caffeine, nicotine, and alcohol close to bedtime
- Create a calming bedtime routine
- Create a relaxing sleep environment
- Have a consistent sleep schedule
- Avoid screens before bed
- Keep electronic devices at a distance from your bed, including cell phones, tablets, and computers.
- Don't do chair yoga or any exercise at night.

Create a Relaxing Sleep Environment

Among all the tips listed above, people might confuse creating a relaxing sleep environment with establishing a calming bedtime routine, such as reading a book, playing soothing music, or using herbal oils. They are tools that can help people relax, unlike the physical environment. So, I'll elaborate on creating a relaxing sleep environment.

Regulate Your Room Temperature

Body temperature, room temperature, and sleep are more closely related than most people realize. Many people try to keep their bedrooms (and beds) as warm as possible because they are cozy, especially in cold winter. But that might be hindering your sleep.

Again, there is no "perfect" sleeping temperature - it varies from person to person. Science found that the ideal room temperature for sleep is around 65 degrees Fahrenheit (18.3 degrees Celsius). The ideal room temperature may vary by a few degrees from person to person, so 65 degrees is a good starting point for experimenting with different thermostat settings to find the optimal temperature for you.

Make Sure Your Room is Dark and Quiet

Our subconscious minds never sleep. While sleeping, your senses continue to receive input and send signals to your brain, where your subconscious processes them. You can wake up when the alarm goes off or if something disturbs your sleep.

By extension, this means that more sensory input leads to a more active mind while you're sleeping, which is why it's so important to have your room as dark and quiet as possible while you're sleeping.

Blackout curtains can help keep outside light out of your bedroom, and turning off electronic devices can further darken the space. Many devices have LEDs that light up when they're charging. If you have any of those devices in your bedroom, remove them from their chargers before bed or charge them in a different room. You can also wear an eye mask to bed if there's still too much light in the room.

If you live in a busy urban area, noise may be a more significant problem. You can try wearing earplugs, but white noise or sound machines are very good at blocking out ambient noise without blocking your ears.

So now you know strategies to eat and sleep better, one more integral part of sustaining your chair yoga routine and long-term wellness is your mindset.

Chapter 11: Shift Your Mindset for Weight Loss Success

Did you know your mindset determines your success in almost every aspect of your life? Having negative self-talk or negative beliefs is normal. Negative beliefs that have brewed over the years make you question whether you can do the chair yoga poses, practice daily, or see any benefit at all.

Our brains function through interconnected neural pathways that can communicate with one another. Scientists used to think these neural pathways could not be changed. In other words, once you see the world one way, it will always be that way. Interestingly, Norman Doidge, M.D., found that our minds can form new neural pathways. The key to this process is positive thought. So, how can we change our mindsets to be more positive?

Techniques for Positive Thinking

Daily Positive Visualization: Visualize positive outcomes— yourself doing every pose with ease and enjoyment. Yes, you can call this daydreaming, but with a specific goal.

Daily Positive Affirmations: Read out loud or silently positive statements regarding you.

Journaling: Write down every small progress you made and pat yourself on the back for completing the routine every day.

Meditation: Clear the noise and chatter in your head and focus on breathing.

Positive Relationships: Socialize with people who have positive energy; avoid or minimize interactions with those who have negative energy.

Channel Emotions Through Creativity: Express your emotions (frustrations or negative thoughts) through coloring books, playing instruments, and other creative hobbies.

Replace Negative Thoughts with Positive Ones: Whenever a negative thought arises, acknowledge it and replace it with a positive one.

Proactively Count Your Blessings: If you frequently count blessings and express gratitude for everything you have, there's simply less room for negative thoughts to sneak in.

What does any of these have to do with chair yoga? Trust me; they can all impact your belief system and help you consistently practice yoga. You can practice one or multiple of them to shape your belief system. You want to be self-aware of negative thoughts and try to neutralize negative thoughts with positive ones.

Unfortunately, many people have way more negative than positive thoughts every minute and every hour. Here are some examples of negative thoughts or self-doubt:

1a) Negative thought: How can I lose weight by doing a few poses while sitting in a chair?

1b) Positive thought: Isn't it amazing that I can lose weight from the comfort of my chair?!

2a) Negative thought: I look awkward when doing chair yoga. I don't want to be laughed at.

2b) Positive thought: What a smart way to get the benefits of yoga by doing a modified version! I'm eager to share it with my friends.

I admit it's not easy to make everything sound positive. To make it easier for you, I've created a list of positive affirmations that you can read or write down daily, whether you first wake up, during the day, or before bedtime. You don't have to come up with positive words yourself; you just need to repeat them in the present tense and believe these words as you read or write them. Then, magic will happen without you knowing how it happened. Shifting your mindset shifts your reality.

Weight Loss Success Affirmations

1. I am committed to making healthy choices for my body.
2. Every day, I'm becoming stronger, healthier, and more confident.
3. I love nourishing my body with wholesome foods.
4. I celebrate each small victory on my weight loss journey.
5. I have the power to change my body and my life.
6. I release old habits and am creating a healthier future.
7. My body is my home, and I am treating it with love and respect.
8. I am patient with myself and take progress one day at a time.
9. I enjoy moving my body and feeling energized.
10. I trust the process and believe in my ability to achieve my weight loss goals.

Chair Yoga Success Affirmations

1. I embrace the gentle and healing practice of chair yoga.
2. My body appreciates the love and care I give it through chair yoga.
3. I am open to flexibility and balance in my life.
4. With each pose, I cultivate inner peace and strength.
5. I honor my body's capabilities and limitations in each practice.
6. I connect deeply with my breath and find tranquility.

7. I am grateful for the support chair yoga provides my wellness journey.

8. My practice deepens with every session, enhancing my well-being.

9. I am present in the moment and find joy in each pose.

10. I honor my commitment to personal growth and self-care through chair yoga.

These affirmations can serve as daily reminders to reinforce positive behavior, increase motivation, and celebrate achievements in both weight loss and chair yoga practices.

You can start your chair yoga session with a positive affirmation or end it with gratitude journaling. You can choose which positive thinking methods that work best for your personality and lifestyle. The bottom line is keeping a positive mindset for long-term fitness success.

Chapter 12: Keep the Body Moving

Now that you have learned 22 simple and effective chair yoga weight loss poses, 10 stretching and relaxation yoga poses, and tips on fueling your body with quality nutrients, controlling cravings, increasing metabolism, getting better sleep, and shifting your mindset for success, you are well-equipped for a successful weight loss journey!

Why Keep Moving?

The CDC recommends that seniors aim for 150 minutes of moderate-intensity aerobic activity (such as brisk walking) per week, but remember, this is a long-term goal. Every small step counts—whether it's 10 minutes of chair yoga or a short stroll around the house, consistency matters more than hitting big numbers right away. Start at a pace that feels comfortable, and celebrate your progress as you gradually build toward this goal.

For example, do 10 minutes of chair yoga daily, then take a 20-minute walk outside to get some fresh air and enjoy the outdoor environment. Or extend your chair yoga to 20 minutes a day, then take a 10-minute brisk walk. You can choose the combination of activities that works best for you.

Easy Ways to Keep Moving Daily

If walking in a park or your neighborhood daily is not feasible due to weather, traffic, or something else, here are some tips to keep your body moving throughout the day.

Increase standing time. Stand up while reading, talking on the phone, or folding laundry.

Fidget while sitting. Move or flex your legs every so often.

Use stairs if available. Walk up and down your stairs (if applicable).

Move during leisure time. Walk around your home when listening to music or podcasts.

Break up screen time. Stand up every 10 minutes when watching TV.

Tidy up your space. Cleaning and organizing your home get you moving while being productive.

Staying mobile can help you create more calorie deficit for weight loss, reduce health risks, and connect the mind and body. Of course, your consistency in practicing chair yoga enables you to be more mobile. As you become more mobile, you can take on more challenging chair yoga poses, where movement becomes both easier and more rewarding over time.

Conclusion

Congratulations on completing this guide! I hope you have found joy and inspiration in our journey together through the 22 essential chair yoga poses for weight loss, the invigorating 14-Day Challenge, and the valuable physical and mental wellness tips provided. With these tools and holistic strategies, you're well-equipped to support your weight loss goals while enhancing mobility, flexibility, energy, and confidence.

As you continue to practice these 22 poses, you can expect to feel revitalized and notice tangible results in the weeks ahead. Embrace the joy and benefits of incorporating the exercises and mindfulness techniques from this book into your daily routine, and let them become lifelong habits.

Remember to celebrate every milestone, no matter how small, and maintain a positive mindset throughout your journey. I am grateful to have been part of your weight loss and wellness experience. I am confident that these practices will lead to a transformative change in your life. Keep practicing, keep smiling, and enjoy the lasting benefits of your dedication and effort.

If this book has helped you, I'd be grateful if you could leave a rating/ review on Amazon. Your support can help others looking for guidance and inspiration, just like you. **Simply scan the QR code below and leave your rating/review now!**

Thank you again for allowing me to be a part of your wellness journey.

Kate M. Right

P.S. If you'd like to gain additional resources and insights to enrich your health and wellness journey, feel free to explore more of my books on physical, mental, and emotional wellness at **harmonybookpublishing.com**.

References

Right, Kate. (2023, November 24). Weight Loss Hacks for Women Over 40: Feel Lighter and More Energetic Starting Week 1. https://www.amazon.com/dp/B0CP1BP6QL

Hawthorne, Aurora (2025, April 15). Simplified Herbal Remedies for Beginners: Natural DIY Solutions for Immune Boost, Stress Relief, Insomnia, Pain Management, Heart Health, Gut Health, Weight Loss, and Lifelong Wellness. https://www.amazon.com/dp/B0F5HKKNS2

Right, Kate. (2024, January 7). Productivity Transformation in 7 Days: Life-Changing Hacks to Shift Your Mindset, Create Priorities, Boost Efficiency, Reduce Stress, and Achieve Work-Life Bliss. https://www.amazon.com/Productivity-Transformation-Days-Life-Changing-Priorities/dp/B0CRRMGLJ2/

Mayo Clinic. (2025, January 25). Nutrition and Healthy Eating. https://www.mayoclinic.org/healthy-lifestyle/nutrition-and-healthy-eating/in-depth/add-antioxidants-to-your-diet/art-20546814

Connected, S. (2023, September 15). More Exercise Doesn't Always Burn More Calories. Science Connected Magazine. Retrieved November 20, 2023, from https://magazine.scienceconnected.org/2021/03/more-exercise-doesnt-always-burn-more-calories/#

Renaissance Village (2023, April 29). Benefits of Antioxidants for Seniors. https://www.renaissancevillages.com/2023/04/benefits-of-antioxidants-for-seniors/

Newsome, Rob and DeBanto, John. (2023, September 19). Aging and Sleep. https://www.sleepfoundation.org/aging-and-sleep

National Institute on Aging. (2025, February 6). Sleep and Older Adults. https://www.nia.nih.gov/health/sleep/sleep-and-older-adults

Smith, Melinda M.A. and Robinson, Lawrence. (2025, January 16). Aging and Sleep. https://www.helpguide.org/aging/healthy-aging/how-to-sleep-well-as-you-age

CDC. (n.d.). Older Adult Activity: An Overview. https://www.cdc.gov/physical-activity-basics/guidelines/older-adults.html

Yale Medicine. (n.d.). Blood Clots in Veins, Heart and Lungs. https://www.yalemedicine.org/conditions/blood-clots-in-veins-heart-and-lungs

St-Onge, M., & Gallagher, D. (2010). Body composition changes with aging: The cause or the result of alterations in metabolic rate and macronutrient oxidation? Nutrition, 26(2), 152–

155. Retrieved November 20, 2023, from
https://www.ncbi.nlm.nih.gov/pmc/articles/PMC2880224/

Yadav, Niva. (2024, May 21). What is Himalayan pink salt and does 'nature's Mounjaro' really help with weight loss? The Standard.
https://www.standard.co.uk/lifestyle/wellness/himalayan-pink-salt-weight-loss-recipe-b1228824.html

Made in United States
Cleveland, OH
10 July 2025

18443731R00079